CBD FOR IBD

The Benefits and Uses of CBD for Inflammatory Bowel Disease

By Elizabeth Tebb

An important note: This book is not intended as a substitute for the medical recommendation of physicians or other health-care providers. Rather, it is intended to offer information to help the reader cooperate with physicians and health professionals in a mutual quest for optimum well-being.
The publisher and the author are not responsible for any goods and/or services offered or referred to in this book and expressly disclaim all liability in connection with the fulfillment of orders for any such goods and/or services and for any damage, loss, or expense to person or property arising out of or relating to them.

CBD For IBD
The Benefits and Uses Of CBD For Inflammatory Bowel Disease
By Elizabeth Tebb

1. Nonfiction:Health & Fitness -Alternative Therapies
2. Nonfiction:Health & Fitness -Diseases -Immune & Autoimmune

ISBN: 9798647089045

Cover design by Elizabeth Tebb

Printed in the United States of America

Independently Published

DISCLAIMER

No part of this publication may be reproduced or transmitted in any form or by any means, mechanical or electronic, including photocopying or recording, or by any information storage and retrieval system, or transmitted by email without permission in writing from the publisher.

While all attempts have been made to verify the information provided in this publication, neither the author nor the publisher assumes any responsibility for errors, omissions, or contrary interpretations of the subject matter herein.

This book is for educational purposes only. The views expressed are those of the author alone and should not be taken as expert instruction or commands. The reader is responsible for his or her own actions.

Adherence to all applicable laws and regulations, including international, federal, state, and local governing professional licensing, business practices, advertising, and all other aspects of doing business in the United States, Canada, or any other jurisdiction is the sole responsibility of the purchaser or reader.

Neither the author nor the publisher assumes any responsibility or liability whatsoever on the behalf of the purchaser or reader of these materials.

Any perceived slight of any individual or organization is purely unintentional.

FORWARD

In 1994, I was diagnosed with ulcerative colitis. Over the course of the next seventeen years of my life, I managed symptoms with a combination of maintenance medications and dietary changes. However, by the spring of 2011 it had become apparent, after trips to the emergency room for pain and dehydration, that the only course of action left to me was to totally remove my large intestine.

In June of 2011, the colon came out and an ileostomy loop was created, leaving part of my rectum attached for later j-pouch creation. This was one of the worst experiences of my life, both physically and emotionally. I had irreparably altered the very anatomy of my body and I was unprepared for the wearing on my mentality that months of recuperation would take, only to repeat the process three months later when my ileostomy was reversed.

Aside from the urgency and loss of motility, I was hopeful that I had made a new start. A couple of bowel obstructions, hemorrhoids, and pouchitis early on taught me the new limits of my body and signs to look for that my j-pouch was functioning below optimum levels. And to handle the day-to-day struggle of pain and scar tissue that affected my ability to move about with ease, I was often prescribed pain medications and muscle relaxants that came with their own side effects.

Added to the stress of my surgeries was the diagnosis of Hashimoto's Disease, another autoimmune disease characterized as hypothyroidism, which presented as continuous hives and exhaustion just over a year after my total colectomy. Suddenly, I was often arthritic, especially in my hands, and forever tired both from the underactive thyroid and multiple trips to the bathroom at night.

But, it wasn't until I after my wedding in 2017 that I even used CBD products at all. Before this, I had maybe tried marijuana a couple of times and found that it wasn't for me. But even so, I was desperate to try a more natural approach to controlling some of the symptoms a "bad day" would have, so that I could participate in activities I enjoyed, or simply get a good night's sleep.

It was on a trip to visit my sister in Colorado that my husband and I attempted CBD products, visiting a dispensary outside of Denver. We discussed uses of CBD and the best forms to use with the staff, comparing products with different ratios of THC to CBD. All told, we left there with about $100 worth of product in the form of edibles, tinctures, and vaporizer.

The next few days, as we explored Boulder or went on a typical "Liz and Alberto Beer Tour" that was a tradition of any of our travels, I experimented with our various CBD products to find a particular product that offered me relief from the symptoms I generally associate with travel: anxiety, increased urgency, stomach cramping, and frequent bathroom trips. Since finding a bathroom in a completely new place can be terrifying if you suffer from IBD, I'm sure you understand how simply worrying about it can become a self-fulfilling prophecy.

It took about a week of careful experimentation and incredibly specific note-taking to realize that what I was benefitting from was rarely a "high" that I chased for the fun of it. Instead, I noticed a general increase in positive thinking and sleep, as well as a decrease in nightly accidents or trips to the bathroom.

In 2019, I started to notice that my routines were no longer keeping the more unpleasant symptoms at bay, and four months into attempting to get pregnant, I developed a pouch-vaginal fistula. I was terrified. No one had ever told me such a thing existed, and even my own research turned up only surgery as a possible treatment option. And so, I had first one, then another failed attempt at a fistulotomy. By November of 2019, I had spent a year battling pain, urgency, and now a fistula with no end in sight.

Finally, my gastroenterologist and surgeon made slight implications that the fistula was simply a secondary issue, caused by something else that was also responsible for the overall decline in my quality of life. After several tests and procedures, as well as a second opinion, in early 2020 my doctors finally agreed that:

1. I had Crohn's Disease
2. I was in j-pouch failure, due to a stricture (narrowing) in the pouch
3. The only way to fix both the stricture and fistula would be to reverse my j-pouch and wear an ostomy for six to nine months, before attempting to fix the fistula. Pardon, fistulas. I developed another one between October 2019 and March 2020.

I was overwhelmed. I'd spent most of my life with one type of Inflammatory Bowel Disease, removed pieces of my myself in an attempt to "cure" it, only to have the other major type? What was more, I had had a total of four surgeries in nine years, all of which seemed to be apparent failures. I was beside myself.

In between all of these procedures, all during my ordeal with Remicade and introduction to Humira, my only escape from the now almost daily discomfort of eating food and constantly using the bathroom, was CBD. It was my solution when the urgency persisted.

I realized then, that had I known of its beneficial effects prior to surgery in 2011, I might have been able to control my UC symptoms long enough to deter its spread. What was more, it was far and away the best treatment for long-term pain I'd tried, with the least consequential side effects. It did not interfere with any other drugs or supplements I needed to take, and was able to control much of my anxiety and depression as I struggled to find a routine that I could manage.

With so much information available about common medications and treatments for IBD, as well as diets that promoted well-being for those who suffer from UC or Crohn's, I realized that the same could not be said for the potential implications of incorporating CBD into the overall treatment plan of patients looking for symptom relief and opportunities to either achieve or retain remission.

Having told you all of this, I compiled this book as one patient seeking to advise others. By no means do I believe that I can tell you with certainty how you should live. Only you can determine the best course for your wellness. However, I hope that in learning of my struggles and experiences, you can see a little of yourself in my story so that, perhaps, you can use what I have learned to reduce or eliminate some of the suffering I have endured for yourself.

I wish you health and luck.

Introduction

The purpose of this book is to review current treatments for managing the symptoms of Inflammatory Bowel Disease (IBD), as well as how CBD can help maintain or even supplement the use of them. By understanding exactly what CBD does in the body, you may find that there are symptoms it can help to alleviate, either intermittently as these symptoms occur or for use over a long period of time during times that your disease is active. In treating chronic conditions such as either ulcerative colitis or Crohn's Disease, CBD can help patients achieve remission in conjunction with medication, or help to maintain longer periods of time without any active symptoms during remission.

Inflammatory Bowel Disease is defined by the CDC (Center for Disease Control) as a "term for two conditions (Crohn's disease and ulcerative colitis) that are characterized by chronic inflammation of the gastrointestinal (GI) tract. Prolonged inflammation results in damage to the GI tract." As will be discussed, there is no cure for either condition, so the best a patient can hope for is long-lasting remission, during which there is no activity in the affected areas of the patient's body and the patient is able to live a typical lifestyle. Remission is any length of time, during which a patient experiences no activity of symptoms.

The CDC reported in 2015 that at the time, approximately 1.3% of the U.S. adult population had been diagnosed with a type of Inflammatory Bowel Disease. Though diagnosis of either type has been increasing in younger populations, the incidence of occurrence is projected to be only about 10% of all reported cases. Onset can begin at any time, though is most commonly diagnosed during puberty and in adults in their mid-thirties and forties. In Crohn's Disease, this is more common than ulcerative colitis, which is less likely to follow any specific age pattern, except in cases of familial correlation.

If you are reading this book, chances are that you or someone you care about has been diagnosed with Inflammatory Bowel Disease. If so, you've probably already found a gastroenterologist and undergone several diagnostic procedures to confirm this. Even at the point of actively seeking a diagnosis, you've already been suffering for far too long. In fact, many patients report waiting months for their doctor to determine the condition causing their symptoms. Others report that they were misdiagnosed and treated for the wrong condition at first. While there are several reasons why this can occur, which I'll include in Chapter 1, all IBD patients have suffered through the symptoms without proper treatment at one point or another.

The fact is that both Crohn's Disease and ulcerative colitis are debilitating and chronic. Whether you're awaiting further testing to receive your diagnosis or you've been coping with the disease for decades, there will always be periods of active symptoms that prevent you from living life. The disease can sometimes seem unpredictable, making it difficult to plan activities or events where you may fear having limited bathroom access. Additionally, the disease can affect your overall wellness in ways that make you more susceptible to malnutrition, fatigue, and a weakened immune system, that can all impact your quality of life.

Some days are going to be bad. Many patients report being unable to work or even leave the house on their worst days during a flare, and the longer the flare continues, the more serious the repercussions that has on your entire body. Keeping all of this in mind, there are many who have reported benefits in using CBD products.

As I outline and discuss the nature of the disease, as well as its treatments, I will touch on systems in the body that contribute to the symptoms you experience. In knowing how Crohn's Disease and ulcerative colitis operate, you'll be more informed about the reactions taking place in your body and what CBD can do to interrupt or negate these reactions, leading to a lessening or even disappearance of certain symptoms.

Please understand that CBD alone, like any other holistic approach, cannot fully manage either disease alone due to the nature of IBD's progression through the body. Indeed, 11% of Crohn's patients will have chronic symptoms, or symptoms that never fully resolve, and up to three-quarters will eventually need some sort of surgery, according to a Healthline overview of treatments. In ulcerative colitis patients, the total removal of the large intestine has been in recent decline as more treatments have become available, but will still become medically necessary for about 32% of UC patients (American Journal of Gastroenterology, 2012). Again, in instances where surgery is recommended, CBD is simply not going to help, and in fact may complicate things for patients who are currently awaiting surgery. It is not recommended that you try introducing CBD into your routine until you have fully healed from surgery.

Another thing to consider is your current age and years that you have lived with IBD. Little research has been conducted on the effects of CBD in people under the age of 18 for certain ethical reasons, and it is unknown if CBD can harm the brain's development. If you are older than 18, you may be able to use CBD. However, I recommend serious discussion with your doctor and careful consideration if you are under the age of 25, as using CBD may not be an approach you should necessarily consider if other treatments have not been exhausted. This can also be true within one year of your diagnosis. Until you have been stable on maintenance drugs, I do not suggest using CBD in any way, as it may impact your body's response to medications and therefore, decrease their effectiveness in the future.

Whether you suffer from mild, moderate, or severe activity of your disease, this book will give you the information you need to make decisions about using CBD for the management of some of these symptoms. While reading, take note of the benefits that CBD can offer in controlling the symptoms you experience, and consider the comparisons in using CBD as opposed to other choices. Before you use any specific regimen or product, carefully consider what you want to use the CBD to control before discussing this with your doctor.

Use this book to determine if you currently experience any of the symptoms discussed in the following chapters. If you do, you may be thinking about using CBD because you want to control either the symptoms themselves, the amount of maintenance medication your doctor has prescribed, or your use of other drugs for the onset of symptoms that carry their own side effects. Whatever your specific reasons, CBD may be able to help!

Chapter One

Understanding IBD

To begin, it is important that you understand there is nothing you specifically did that led to your diagnosis, nor could there be any guarantee that a change in your lifestyle could have prevented your diagnosis. Though as yet the exact cause of Inflammatory Bowel Disease is unknown, it is thought to be the cause of a conjunction of risk factors. Though anyone can be diagnosed with either Crohn's Disease or ulcerative colitis at any time, their rates of incidence among certain populations seem to play a role in your overall risk assessment.

Genetic Factors

Both Crohn's Disease and ulcerative colitis are thought to be related to specific genes found more prevalently in particular populations. Though both conditions appear to affect men and women equally, there is a larger rate of incidence among those with Caucasian and Ashkenazi descent. Among families, the child of a patient with either condition has a 10% likelihood of later diagnosis, and about 20% of patients have another close family member with IBD (Tresca, 2020). This seems to suggest that at least in part, inherited DNA markers are likely either indicators of risk or themselves the causes of both conditions.

Where there is a familial link, the patient is more likely to be diagnosed at a younger age, and in Crohn's Disease, may suggest the severity of symptoms that lead to surgery (Journal of Crohn's and Colitis, 2018). The National Human Genome Research Institute (NHGRI) presented findings in 2015 of their explanation of autoimmune risk assessment by stating the following:

"Genetic studies have shown that people with autoimmune diseases possess unique genetic variants, but most of the alterations are found in regions of the DNA that do not carry genes. Scientists have suspected that the variants are in DNA elements called enhancers, which act like switches to control gene activities."

These super enhancers, or SEs, seem to control the communication between certain areas of the brain and the immune system. Researchers at the National Human Genome Research Institute "identified several hundred [SEs], and further analysis showed that they largely control the activities of genes that encode cytokine and cytokine receptors. These types of molecules are important for T cell function because they enable them to communicate with other cells and to mount an immune response" (2016). It seems likely that further research into identifying these super enhancers in our genetics will eventually lead to individualized gene therapy to retrain our immune systems, but for now, their role in our risk assessment, like that of c-reactive proteins, is to identify that there is a likely risk of autoimmunity.

Environmental Factors

It has thus been established that while there are specific genetic variants that seem inherent to autoimmunity, these variants do not directly affect any particular part of the human body. Therefore, the enhancers (or DNA elements known as SEs) found among patients diagnosed with an autoimmune disease must be activated in a particular region in the body that leads to a certain diagnosis. Gene activity in the joints will lead to Rheumatoid Arthritis, while this same activity in the digestive tract (esophagus down to the rectum) will lead to IBD, the type depending on the location and nature of inflammation.

However, much about the interactions between environment and genetics is unknown. "Previous studies have demonstrated concordance in age at diagnosis, disease location and behaviour, and need for IBD-related surgery in affected family members, but have been limited by small sample sizes and lack of examination of the genetics or microbial composition underlying such phenotypes" (Journal of Crohn's and Colitis, 2018). This raises the question: were we doomed to develop our condition because of a deficiency in the gut micro biome we have been exposed to since birth?

According to a study published by "Gut" in 2013, an imbalance in the composition of the gut micro biome and reaction of other cells to the gut microbiota may be primary indicators of Inflammatory Bowel Disease, both being present in association with IBD. The foods we eat may interact with our gut in such a way as to contribute to inflammation. This is completely supported by the fact that the highest rates of incidence are almost exclusively in first-world nations, where diets contain more refined or processed ingredients and larger amounts of certain foods. "Specifically, the introduction of the Western diet (which is high in fat and protein and low in fruits and vegetables) has been proposed as an explanation for the increase in IBD incidence" in these countries, claims one study in the journal Gastroenterology and Hepetology (2015).

Current research suggests that, "autoimmune diseases are most prevalent in highly industrialized nations but rare in less developed countries" (Fakhoury et al., 2014). This points to a major difference in the environments we are exposed to and the bacteria that live in them, in addition to possible dietary links. Possibly, an imbalance in the gut micro biome is caused by the over-sterilization of our environments as we grow from babies. Essentially, our guts lack a variety of flora because developed nations tend to sanitize and clean any and all objects a baby might touch.

Again, it is impossible to know how much our genetics predispose us to developing an autoimmune disease. As of now, there are no genetic tests that could be done either to measure the risk assessment of inherited autoimmunity before conception or your child's likelihood of developing autoimmunity through blood tests or amniocentesis while in vitro. Likewise, there is no way to plan for a balanced environment of bacteria through which you can decrease your child's likelihood of future diagnosis. This is where a third component may also come into play, and is itself a part of our environments that may tend to support both a family link and a correlation to the "enhancers" that interact with our guts.

Stress Factors

One particular variable in understanding the impact of our environments on our disease is stress. On a very chemical level, this is due to our body's natural production of cortisol, a stress hormone that creates inflammation. This seems to be key in understanding sudden relapses in symptoms of both Crohn's Disease and ulcerative colitis, which can occur even without any other significant changes to diet or medication during periods of prolonged difficulty.

But stress is more than just a vehicle for activating symptoms after a period of remission. It is more widely believed to be related to the conditions under which a patient's condition is first "triggered." Triggers are important in understanding what caused your symptoms to begin, and will be discussed further in a moment, but it is crucial in understanding IBD that stress be given credence as part of our overall risk factor in the development and treatment of our disease.

In a 2005 article written in "Gut," it is posited that stress responses in the body directly interact with the immune system, both systemically and locally. Says the article, "environmental factors which trigger initial presentation and subsequent relapses, and the mechanisms by which they act, are less clearly understood. Psychological stress is one environmental factor which has long been anecdotally reported as having a relationship with activity in IBD." Therefore, it is likely that autoimmunity first develops during a period of prolonged stress on the body, in which cortisol is overproduced and causes unnecessary inflammation.

This certainly explains the age ranges during which most IBD patients first experience symptoms. As I've mentioned, Crohn's Disease in particular seems to be diagnosed during the ages of 15 to 25, and again between 35 and 45, with a peak after 50 as well (Tresca, 2020). These ages follow prolonged periods of stress on the human body caused by changes in hormones.

From 15 to 25, both boys and girls undergo puberty. The shift in hormones causes moodiness, acne breakouts, and all the normal ups and down of settling into the person you're going to be. From 35 to 45, both men and women might feel stressed to perform well at work and engage in stressful life events. For example, buying a house or relocating are huge life events that do not resolve quickly. In addition, women are more likely to be pregnant at least once during this time, which is a stress on the body both physically and hormonally. After the age of 50, both men and women will experience a decline in hormone levels, and women will experience menopause.

If you are like me, and you were not diagnosed at a time when you underwent physical stress, then maybe you too suffer from depression and anxiety. Neither directly cause our condition, but it has been widely argued that those with autoimmune conditions are more susceptible to these disorders. The 2005 study published in "Gut" made a correlation between these conditions and Inflammatory Bowel Disease, saying, "in addition to immunosuppression, chronic psychological stress has also been shown to be associated with subclinical increases in inflammation." In fact, the study cited clusters of patients with a wide range of indicators that also correlate to stress, finding that those with clinical depression or heart conditions caused by stress were more vulnerable to autoimmune responses in general.

This is not to say that simply reducing stress in your life would have helped you avoid your diagnosis, though it is always a good idea to do so. The changes your body undergoes throughout life are unavoidable, and this factor simply points to the reason why the disease occurs most frequently during these ages. Though the initial onset of symptoms may begin during these stressful milestones in our lives, there is one final factor which may influence your overall risk assessment in developing Inflammatory Bowel Disease.

Triggers

As I've stated, we were genetically predisposed towards autoimmunity, and our environments facilitated interactions between our immune systems and guts. More probably, environmental stressors are responsible for that "switch" to be flipped in our DNA enhancers, thereby activating the onset of symptoms as the wrong message is communicated to our immune system. When this occurs, our otherwise normally functioning body accidentally unlearns a fundamental lesson.

The immune system is responsible for identifying and fighting external agents that our body treats as harmful. Therefore, it must know the difference between "self" and "other" in order to do its job. When our immune cells "forget" a part of "self," we develop our disease. The National Human Genome Institute has conducted research into the Super Enhancers (SEs) that appear in the DNA variants of patients with autoimmune diseases, as "a large number of disease-associated genetic alterations were found to fall within SEs, suggesting that disease occurs when these switches malfunction."

The malfunction in these switches is often referred to as the "trigger." This could have been something you ate, a medication that you took (there is currently research being conducted into correlations between the over-prescribing of antibiotics, for example, or in predisposed people who are prescribed Accutane), the development of another condition, or a stressful life event. Most patients can trace the start of their symptoms back to a specific occurrence.

Remember, whether you took a medication that a doctor prescribed or sat down and ate three bowls of Raisin Bran one day (or was that just me?), no one could have foreseen that any one event would flip this switch inside of us. However, in understanding the complicated relationship between our environments, our genetics, and our stress levels, I hope I can at least educate you on our primary concern when thinking of ways to both reduce the symptoms of IBD themselves as well as the catalyst behind the relapse of symptoms. Moving forward, stress will become a topic as we think of ways that CBD may benefit our condition.

Chapter Two
Symptoms of IBD

Now that you're a little more familiar with some of the "why" of Inflammatory Bowel Disease, let's review some of the "how" with this condition. As I go through major signs and symptoms of both Crohn's Disease and ulcerative colitis, take notes on the ones that you experience most, taking time to think about when these symptoms occur and to what degree.

Where it is appropriate to mention them, I'll also cover some of the secondary symptoms of IBD. These are things we might experience as a result of a symptom of IBD, though not in itself a sign that you are suffering from IBD. Many of these might might be serious, however, and worth noting as you take stock of how your condition affects you. It is possible to address some of these with the use of CBD.

As with any condition, we experience some or all of these symptoms in our own way. This might be only during a flare, or occasionally in remission. This might be daily, or only on a "bad day." The more observant you are of the patterns in your symptoms, the more you'll be able to fine tune the use of CBD as a part of your treatment plan, as well as what types of products might work best.

Abdominal Cramping And Pain

Most of us will experience horrible stomach pains, either after eating, just before needing to use the bathroom, or while going to the bathroom. It might be all three. The reason we feel such intense cramping is because as we eat, we signal to our brains that it's time to move things along. Then, as food moves through our intestines, it scrapes against the areas of inflammation inside.

Especially in patients who suffer from proctitis, or inflammation of the lining of the rectum, this pain is felt just prior to or during bowel movements, as the pain in the rectum radiates upwards. The Mayo Clinic estimates that approximately 30% of patients with IBD experience proctitis. Though this is more common with ulcerative colitis, patients with CD may also suffer from this.

In patients with left-sided, right-sided, or pancolitis, this pain may be more constant, like menstrual cramps, ebbing and flowing throughout the day. In patients with Crohn's, this same pain may be present in the small intestine, which is just around the area of your belly button. It may worsen after eating, but may be present on its own, during periods of intermittent fasting or between meals. Be aware of this pain and whether it worsens when you eat, exercise, move a certain way, or stand or sit for long periods.

Your abdomen may be tender to the touch. This is more common with Crohn's, but can affect those with moderate to severe UC as well. This might also be a sign of an obstruction, and it is important that you monitor this tenderness.

Urgency

Whether because you actually need to go or not, the feeling of needing to go is a common symptom of Inflammatory Bowel Disease. This is called tenesmus. A study conducted in collaboration with the Crohn's and Colitis Foundation found that in UC patients reporting their symptoms, the most prevalent symptom reported was an urgency to use the bathroom (IBD Journal, 2020). This can make going out or traveling very stressful. Before my Crohn's diagnosis, I felt chained to my house. The idea of being trapped on a bus in the Lincoln Tunnel on my way into the city terrified me, and I'd often refuse to make plans or find a way out of them in order to avoid the possibility of having an accident.

Secondary symptoms associated with this feeling can include fissures and hemorrhoids as a result of straining to go. These can also impact the quality of life (QOL) that a patient is capable of during a flare. Even those of us who don't suffer from depression or anxiety may have symptoms associated with these disorders simply by trying to handle the urges of their bodies in social or professional settings.

Frequency

In conjunction with urgency, frequency is often reported as a symptom of both Crohn's and colitis, though it is possible for many to struggle to pass stool even when they feel the need. The Mayo Clinic lists diarrhea as a common symptom of both UC and Crohn's, citing persistence and severity of the symptom as the most debilitating of both conditions, as its secondary symptoms can greatly impact a person's overall health very easily.

Many secondary symptoms can crop up due to frequency. For example, water retention or nutrient absorption can be greatly diminished when patients are constantly producing liquid stool. It can be easy to become dehydrated or feel weak and dizzy. A patient might have significant drops in their blood pressure.

Blood Or Mucus In Stool

If you do use the bathroom and notice blood (red tinge, clumps caused by clots, or smears when wiping) or mucus (white streaks, light specks in stool), just know that this is a hallmark of ulcerative colitis, though less commonly of Crohn's (Fakhoury, 2014). Due to the inflammation in your intestines, your body may form polyps, accesses, or ulcers along the lining which can weep blood. The mucus that is naturally produced in the rectum can be shed alarmingly. Researchers have noted that "human studies have demonstrated that IBDs, such as Crohn's disease, are characterized by a defect in the epithelial barrier and altered mucus production, leading to an increase in intestinal permeability and toxins adherence in the intestinal cells" (Fakhoury, 2014). Therefore, as the barrier of our digestive lining is constantly worn away, both blood and mucus can become visible in stool.

If you do have several bloody stools a day, you may be at risk for anemia, which can leave you feeling weak and shaky. When I was twelve, my mom became suspicious that my remission was over when I started coming home from school and sleeping. In fact, anemia is the single most predictive symptom of revisits to the ER among Crohn's patients or to the necessity of a total colectomy among UC patients, according to different studies published during the same month in the Journal of Crohn's and Colitis (January, 2020).

Nausea And Vomiting

Though often not a direct symptom of Inflammatory Bowel Disease, nausea and vomiting can both occur in either Crohn's Disease or ulcerative colitis. This is more common in Crohn's Disease, where inflammation of the mucosa throughout the digestive tract can affect a patient's appetite. The Crohn's and Colitis Foundation notes that changes in appetite may be a sign that the progression of either condition may be worsening. Mild symptoms of Crohn's and colitis rarely involve vomiting, so if there is no other reason for this symptom except a relapse in your condition, contact your doctor to determine if your medication is either causing this or failing to control your disease as it flares.

The feeling of nausea can occur also as a result of treatment for IBD. Biologics such as Humira, Remicade, Entyvio, Stelara, or Simponi are often combined with the chemical citrate in loading doses, which are already quite strong in order to deter the development of antibodies the first and second time you receive these treatments. Talk with your doctor about your nausea if you suspect that your biologic is causing you to feel nauseous. You may not tolerate citrate well, and can receive treatments without this additive if necessary. The most important factor here is that you control the damage that vomit does, by eroding the lining of your esophagus and damaging the enamel of your teeth.

Nausea and vomiting can also be a sign of bowel obstruction, which can happen as a result of active inflammation or narrowing in the mucosa of the intestines. This is more common in Crohn's Disease. Though patients with UC can still experience nausea or vomiting as a result of eating foods that trigger symptoms, obstructions are less likely to be the true cause. If you believe you have vomited as a result of an obstruction in the digestive tract, it is important to visit an emergency room for care.

In addition, recent abdominal surgery for your IBD increases your risk of obstruction. This is in part due to the complexity of passing food very quickly through a shortened amount of intestine, as well as because much of the flesh is still inflamed and healing following your procedure. I have personally been hospitalized for three obstructions, two of them within six weeks of my first and second steps of j-pouch surgery. The third one really should have been a clue that I had Crohn's Disesase.

Exhaustion And Weakness

Feeling tired or feeling weak is rarely indicative of any specific malady, but many patients suffering from an autoimmune disease identify these feelings *despite* getting a good night's sleep. In fact, depending on the severity of symptoms, this can be one of the most challenging parts of Inflammatory Bowel Disease, as many patients find they often do not have the energy to participate in any kind of activity, which simply creates a vicious cycle of feeling weak and slowly causing your body to weaken.

There are several reasons why a patient may be tired, and it's important to understand them in order to plan for and address exhaustion appropriately. First, the feeling of weakness or exhaustion rarely has any link to the amount of physical activity or sleep that you've had. In fact, the feelings can linger even if you sleep a full night and remain sedentary throughout the day. Nothing you have done or could do will improve these feelings until the underlying cause is addressed.

A secondary cause of these feelings is tied to how often you use the bathroom. Especially if you get up during the night because of your condition, you may be interrupting your sleep pattern. Anemia caused by frequent, bloody stools will add to these feelings as well, so communicate often with your doctor during a flare about these feelings in order to determine how you can treat these secondary symptoms by supplementing valuable nutrients that you may be losing.

Vitamin Deficiency

The depletion of certain vitamins from your body may also cause feelings of tiredness. You can ask your doctor to check your vitamin levels to determine if you need to supplement your intake of fat soluble vitamins such as iron, vitamin D, vitamin B6 and B12, and potassium. Since fat soluble vitamins take the longest to absorb in our digestive tract, any inflammation or ulceration may render us deficient in these nutrients, many of which can also affect our energy levels.

If you have had surgery to remove any part of your intestine, this will become even more difficult. You should regularly have a full blood panel completed for signs of vitamin deficiency and make sure to eat lots of foods rich in fat soluble vitamins and minerals. Using multivitamins or other supplements should be discussed with your doctor, as it is possible to ingest toxic levels of these vitamins.

Next Steps

Now that we've reviewed the signs and symptoms that you may be experiencing a flare, or relapse of your disease, it's time to discuss how to use this chapter in your wellness plan.

Download an app: There are several daily tracker applications available specifically for the use of IBD patients, and several other that can be used in any capacity. The goal of your tracker should be to help you begin building the correlation between your symptoms and your routines. This can help you to identify trends in symptoms so you are better able to notice the beginnings of a relapse, identify foods you do not tolerate well, and

what your "normal" is as compared to a flare. Try any one of these:
Cara Care- Designed for IBD and IBS, this tracker lets you track bowel movements, symptoms, food, and stress. You can input your medication to keep track of it daily and make notes of how you feel physically and emotionally. Cara will graph your trends so you can see your data over time.

Colitis Watch- This application let's you input your food and bowel movements, and can also tell you where the nearest bathroom is if you let the app access your location. This is a great app for flares, and over time, it can tell you what foods you generally seem to eat on a good day as well as a bad day, based on your previous logs.

My IBD Care- This tracker allows you to track your general well-being, input medications, and track your sleep patterns. Though the emphasis is not on food, it does track your trends to find correlations between your stress levels and your wellness. It also gives you access to thousands of articles from databases on Inflammatory Bowel Disease, spotlighting things in which you take an interest. This app was designed by gastroenterologists and psychologists, and is great for anyone who is triggered by stress.

myIBD- This app has a huge focus on medical history and even accounts for other medical conditions, for which you may require treatment. Personally, this one is the most comprehensive if you are a sufferer of Multiple Autoimmune Syndrome, which is characterized by the diagnosis of three or more autoimmune conditions. You can input any type of medication, as opposed to only ones used in the treatment of IBD. Food, bowel movements, mood, pain, and history provide data for recognizing trends and supports family sharing for children suffering from IBD.

Try an elimination diet: You may be poised to download an app and begin tracking, but you are in a current flare and everything you input isn't telling you *how* to get better. You purchased this book looking for relief and you're ready to try anything that helps. Well, without knowing what hurts you, you might not be able to do anything more than react to symptoms. CBD might help, but how will you know it's the CBD and not your medication? Let's eliminate the other variables and focus on only the controls: CBD, your food intake, your medications, and your routine. To do this, you might need to try an elimination diet while you experiment with CBD products. Give yourself a week or so of predictable foods to ensure that adding CBD is actually beneficial. Remove everything except a select few foods, trying each food one by one for signs of worsening symptoms. If you fear that gluten, sugar, or dairy is a trigger, try one of those early on to determine if you go more frequently or experience more pain. I like BRAT the most for this (bananas, rice, applesauce, and toast). Even though I hate bananas, this is about controlling symptoms in order to introduce a new thing.

Take stock of your health: This might be plausible using the app of your choice, but it's also really important that you check in with your doctor as well and review recent labs, procedures, and medication changes as well. For CBD to help, you have to know how it's helping. That means knowing if you are in a flare and what medications you are using, at what dosage. Knowing this is important to determine when it is a good idea for you to begin using CBD, because you need to be purposeful in deciding when to start, down to what time of day. If you are comfortable sharing with your doctor your intent to use CBD, do so. By itself, it is not an illegal drug, and can easily be ordered over the internet no matter what your state's current policy on marijuana is. You and your doctor may be able to set a goal together for what you want it to help.

Now that you understand your own symptoms and how you can keep track of them to notice trends in your general wellness, and have spoken with your doctor about your health and your intent, let's dive into your other medications so you can get a picture of the benefits and pitfalls inherent in them, which will help you decide how CBD can be incorporated into your treatment plan.

Chapter Three

Treatments For IBD

You've already been seen by a gastroenterologist, who diagnosed you with either ulcerative colitis or Crohn's Disease. He or she has probably already prescribed a medication to help control the inflammation and may have also suggested changes to your lifestyle that could reduce the chances of symptoms relapsing, or "flaring," as well as curb the severity of the symptoms you experience.

In this chapter, we'll discuss the available treatments for these conditions, as well as benefits and drawbacks to using each. Keep in mind, the goal of your doctor's treatment plan for you is to prescribe the least invasive medication with the most benefit to your quality of life. Whether you have been prescribed a combination or find that you see a vast improvement from diet alone, let's explore how these treatments work to better highlight the ways in which CBD might help.

First, it's important that your doctor has definitively diagnosed you with a type of Inflammatory Bowel Disease. Many other conditions exist that mimic the symptoms of Crohn's and UC, but a diagnosis of "colitis" does not necessarily entail an autoimmune disease. Additionally, those who suffer from Clostridium difficile, or c. diff, may actually cause their case to worsen by using CBD. Make sure you've spoken thoroughly with your doctor at a follow-up after your diagnostic testing to review his or her findings. A good gastroenterologist will have performed many of the following in order to rule out any other cause first:

Blood tests- Markers in the blood may suggest an autoimmune disease, such as white blood count and c-reactive protein levels. Your doctor may also test for vitamin deficiencies or red blood cell count if he or she suspects that you are anemic as a result of rectal bleeding.

Stool Sample- In order to rule out the aggressive bacterial infection known as c. diff, which mimics IBD symptoms, your doctor will need a stool sample. As much as we dislike doing this, IBD is an elimination diagnosis, meaning it's what you have when you don't appear to have any other cause for your symptoms. If you do test positive for c. diff, that doesn't mean you don't have IBD as well, so by itself this test only completes part of the picture. However, in conjunction with a fecal calprotectin test, which measures your body's inflammatory response in the gut, your doctor can begin to connect your symptoms to an autoimmune disease, A positive level will be anything over 100. Your doctor will also be able to detect red blood cells in your stool, confirming that you are bleeding somewhere in your digestive tract.

Imaging Studies- Whether your doctor wants to perform more invasive diagnostics later depends on x-ray, CAT scan, MRI, or barium studies. Though x-ray and CAT scan can only show the outlines of things, they can show enlarging due to inflammation or perforation in extreme cases. For more conclusive results, your doctor will likely order an MRI or barium study with contrast. You'll drink the chalky stuff and have pictures taken of your abdomen every 15 minutes for about an hour, as the liquid moves through your digestive tract. The imaging equipment will see this liquid, which will indicate where the inflammation inside of you is located.

Colonoscopy and Endoscopy- Once your doctor has run other tests that more clearly indicate the part of your digestive tract where you seem to have inflammation, he or she will perform an outpatient procedure in which, using a camera affixed to a flexible tube, your digestive tract is carefully examined for signs of

Crohn's Disease or ulcerative colitis. The endoscopy begins when the scope is inserted down the throat, the colonoscopy begins with the scope inserted through the anus. Though both can be performed conscious or unconscious, one may be preferred or contraindicated given past medical history, toleration of anesthesia, and other underlying conditions.

Once you have your diagnosis, you and your doctor will speak about the extent of current activity, its location, and its severity. If need be, take notes and ask for copies of his or her findings for your own records. If you have an online portal where these reports can be accessed, use them to discuss your symptoms and proposed treatment plans. Let's review what medications and treatment you may be taking or that your doctor believes you should consider next. As we do this, I will mention the benefits and drawbacks of each. Please note, your doctor has prescribed you drugs that he or she believe will be more of a benefit than a harm to you. No drugs, even over the counter drugs, are completely without side effects or contraindications. It is not recommended that you try to control your condition without any medication.

Steroids

In most cases, remission is achieved by aggressively treating a patient with corticosteroids to reduce the body's ability to produce inflammatory processes in the body as well as with maintenance drugs to control the body's overall ability to continue causing symptoms.

Types: Prednisone, prenisolone, budesonide, tixocortol, hydrocortisone acetate, betamethasone, Encort, Uceris

Benefits: Steroids are powerful anti-inflammatories that reduce the inflammation of autoimmune diseases, including Crohn's Disease and ulcerative colitis. Says the Mayo Clinic, "Corticosteroids mimic the effects of hormones your body produces naturally in your adrenal glands, which are small glands that sit on top of your kidneys." When a patient is experiencing a flare, steroids can help to regain control of the symptoms before serious complications can occur. If a flare is caught early enough, a patient can avoid being hospitalized or having surgery when the severity of the illness is mild to moderate. They can also greatly improve arthritic pains, which are typical among all autoimmune diseases. If a patient has recently felt unable or unwilling to eat, either because it causes pain or their appetite has diminished, steroids will increase appetite and cause weight gain.

Drawbacks: Steroids may have many benefits, but they are not meant for long-term care. It is incredibly detrimental to the body to be on steroids for long periods, which is why most doctors will instruct patients to take calcium and vitamin D supplements while on steroids for any length of time. However, while the ability of steroids to leech calcium from the bones is dangerous on its own, osteoporosis is only one of many serious side effects. Steroids can also exacerbate mental or mood disorders. They can exacerbate, or even trigger, diabetes. They can cause cataracts or glaucoma. If you taper your dose too quickly or not all, you could cause severe adrenal deficiency that could be dangerous. It is also important to know that steroids are immunosuppressants, meaning they keep your immune system from fighting off infection. This is an important part of your healing when you suffer from an autoimmune disease, but may make you more prone to catching communicable diseases or developing infections.

Side Effects: increased appetite, weight gain, fluid retention (which can cause "moon face"), increased thirst, mood swings, hyperactivity, insomnia, acne, high blood pressure, fatty lipomas, fluctuations in blood sugar, poor memory or concentration

5-Asa's

5 aminosalicylic acids, or 5-ASA's are often the first family of drugs that doctors prescribe for the long-term treatment of IBD. They work to decrease inflammation in the lining of your intestines. Depending on the area of inflammation, the medication can be taken orally or rectally. It is not meant for severe cases, but is effective in controlling symptoms caused by the abnormal inflammation of your condition, as well as stopping the further spread of your condition to healthy tissue.

Types: mesalamine, sulfasalazine, Azulfidine, Dipentum, Colazal, Asacol, Lialda, Apriso, Pentasa, Mezavant, Salofalk

Benefits: These drugs are relatively mild maintenance medications that have minimal long-term side effects on the body. They can be taken all at once or one at a time throughout the day, to suit the preference of a patient. Though some can be quite costly for the amount of pills required, it is much easier to reduce the doses of these drugs once a patient is in remission, in order to maintain remission. For ulcerative colitis patients with distal proctitis (inflammation in the rectum only), the medication can be taken as a suppository to be directly absorbed by the affected mucosa. It has high rates of effectiveness in mild to moderate cases of ulcerative colitis. One study (Katz et al. 2010) found that, "Overall, 5-ASAs have been proven to achieve remission in approximately 70% of UC patients."

Drawbacks: Sadly, 5-ASA's are not shown to be as effective in Crohn's Disease patients, and are used for mild cases or cases only affecting the rectum with varying degrees of success. Even in UC patients, your doctor may try more than one at a time to maximize its success in controlling your symptoms, which might become very costly. Because mesalamine is commonly branded differently with different strengths, there are no generics that can be substituted. I recently went through my old files, looking for documents that are too old to be kept, and found a receipt for my Lialda in 2010 that was three hundred dollars for a one-month supply. Though I'm sure this was also because it was new at the time, it is often difficult to keep up with the financial drain of these conditions. Another drawback I discovered in this family of drugs was my sulfa allergy, which eliminated a few possible drugs for me early on.

Side Effects: headaches, constipation, nausea, abdominal cramping, kidney problems in rare cases

Immunomodulators

Immunomodulators do exactly what they sound like: they modulate how your body's immune system is able to function. By doing this, these drugs effectively curtail your ability to produce the classic abnormal inflammation that causes the symptoms of Crohn's and colitis. These drugs can also be used concomitantly with biologic therapies.

These drugs were around before most biologics were widely available, and are effective in treating moderate to severe forms of both types of Inflammatory Bowel Disease. Many of these medications have also been used as maintenance medications for certain types of cancer.

Types: 6-meracaptapurine (6-mp), methotrexate (Trexall), azathioprine (Azasan, Imuran), cyclosporine (Gengraf, Neoral, Sandimmune)

Benefits: For both Crohn's Disease and ulcerative colitis, these drugs have an incredibly high success rate. In fact, the success rate of these drugs in 1995 by Pearson et al. was 95%. These same rates of success have been repeatedly upheld by other studies done around the world (Sandborn, et al 2000, Prefontaine et al. 2009). A study of steroid-dependent UC patients found that the introduction of azathioprine or 6-mp allowed the majority to achieve remission (Fraser et al. 2002). In up to 70% of patients, these drugs can help a patient to achieve mucosal healing, with clinical indications that "then we have a strong reason to recommend an earlier and wider use of both immunosuppressants and biological agents, which have clearly demonstrated their ability to induce [mucosal healing]" (Ardizzone, 2010). In UC patients, those that took immunomodulators as compared to those with long-standing and extensive UC, were 3.2 times less likely to develop colon cancer (Beaugerie et al. 2009).

Drawbacks: Unlike 5-ASA's, which can be started any time, these drugs are indicated only once a patient has reached a stage of steroid dependency, which can be characterized by at least two occasions of continuous steroid use at a dose of 15 mg/day in a calendar year or those who tend to relapse within three months of stopping steroids (Ardizzone, 2010). This is quite limiting on a patient's quality of life. Once a patient is on an immunomodulator, it takes time to fully be present in a patient's system. This can mean that patients stay on steroids even longer, suffering from both the adverse effects of those drugs along with those of immunomodulators. A study in the American Journal of Gastroenterology posited that, "Although effective for many patients, these medications are associated with risks, most notably infection and malignancy, with infection occurring far more commonly." There are many other research studies only now being able to track the adverse effects of long-term use of these drugs, finding an increased risk of bone marrow and joint lymphoma and certain skin cancers. More immediately, however, there is an increased risk of opportunistic infection, noted within the first year of use among 2.2% of patients. These medications should also be discussed with your doctor if you become pregnant or plan to become pregnant, as there are serious risks to the development of the fetus.

Side effects: headaches, trouble sleeping, joint pain, pancreatitis, leg cramps, canker sores, rashes, fever, decreased kidney function, birth defects or miscarriage in women, and decreased sperm count in men

Biologics

Biologics are usually intravenous solutions that can be injected through syringe or fed continuously into the bloodstream through infusion. Biologics work in a few ways to reduce your body's ability to produce the inflammation the causes symptoms of both Crohn's Disease and ulcerative colitis. Some work to prevent white blood cells from entering inflamed tissue, but their most effective method of use is in targeting certain pathways that produce cytokines.

Cytokines are part of the immune response, and the job of many is causing inflammation. These proteins are generated along specific pathways that have been mapped in IBD patients, which suggests that the body's inability to recognize homeostasis (the "all is well" status) in the gut is due to misfires along these pathways, "demonstrating that the same cytokine can act on multiple arms of the immune system to promote inflammation" (Knights et al. 2014). The biologics suppress these proteins, even when the pathways from the brain misfire, by blocking the proteins from interacting with their receptors and creating a Th-1 response, which produces the different proteins named above, and instead creates a balance with the Th-2 response. "In contrast, Th2 cells lead to production of anti-inflammatory cytokines" (Fakhoury et al. 2014).

Types: infliximab (Remicade), adalimumab (Humira), go-limumab (Simponi), vedolizumab (Entyvio), and (Stelara)

Benefits: Biologics are not pills you take every day. They are infusions you inject or receive intravenously in your doctor's office. This can be every four to eight weeks in most cases. That may be easier for many patients to handle. In Crohn's patients, moderate to severe symptoms can be controlled within the first three injections, which are typically stronger doses called "loading" doses. Because these drugs are not pills, the intravenous solutions cannot be accidentally forgotten or skipped, which means that your body is steadily in supply of the medication until your next dose.

Drawbacks: These drugs suppress your body's natural immune response in order to discourage overproduction of inflammatory proteins, but this also means you are at further risk for developing infection. While on these drugs, it is not recommended that you receive any live vaccinations and you may want to take extra precautions during the flu season. "As the immune response to vaccination is generally blunted by immunosuppression, the IBD patient should ideally be vaccinated soon after diagnosis before the commencement of immunosuppressive therapy," one study claims (Farraye et al. 2017). Biologics are strong intravenous drugs that were originally designed for use as maintenance chemotherapy drugs, which means you may experience many of the same side effects people associate with chemotherapy in a mild way. There is also an increased risk of developing certain cancers later on. These are certain lymphomas that are associated with autoimmune diseases in general, but that are exacerbated in anti-TNF inhibitors by about 1.8% (Bewtra et al. 2015). Additionally, "the use of anti-TNF for 1 year conferred an almost twofold increased risk for developing [skin melanoma]." If you discontinue these drugs, your body may naturally develop antibodies to the medication, and you cannot take it again. This will increase the likelihood of other drugs in this family to induce similar reactions, so it is important to seek help if you begin to experience symptoms of an allergic reaction, particularly anaphylaxis, if you restart any of these medications.

Side Effects: nausea, vomiting, chills, headaches, rash at injection or IV site, tiredness, weakness, loss of hair, high blood glucose levels

Surgery

In severe cases of IBD, surgery may become necessary to achieve quality of life. Though this looks different in Crohn's Disease than it does in ulcerative colitis, neither will fully "cure" your condition. Remember, your body still believes it is in a state of dysbiosis (out of harmony), and will fight a non-existent threat by causing unwarranted inflammation. However, surgery can remove parts of your intestine where this inflammation has caused irreparable damage, often in cases that prevent or address serious life-threatening consequences such as sepsis, toxic megacolon, perforation, and the development of colon cancer.

The Mayo Clinic estimates that about half of all Crohn's patients will need surgery at some point, and as I've stated earlier, the age of a patient at diagnosis can often indicate this need. Though the rates of incidence for surgery are on a downward trend as anti-TNF drugs are becoming more widely available to patients, abscesses and fistulas may develop that require surgery even in patients who do not indicate the need for resection. Resection may be only segments of intestine, or it may be the entire large intestine. For about 25.4% UC patients, a proctocolectomy will become a necessity by the twenty-year mark, though this rate is as high as 35% (Hwang, 2008). In about 13% of patients, this could be within the first five years of diagnosis (Sunil et al. 2013).

Benefits: Surgery can permanently solve the problem of widespread and severe inflammation where it is limited to only specific areas for Crohn's patients, or to the colon in UC patients. By surgically removing the damaged tissue, you may experience a greater quality of life than you have been able to achieve with medication alone. In the instances where other serious conditions indicate the need for surgery, you may avoid life-threatening repercussions of your condition. In UC patients, this can essentially eliminate the symptoms of the disease, without needing medication for the rest of your life to achieve this. Additionally, colon cancer risks increase with the length of time that you live with the disease, with an 18% risk at the thirty year mark. In Crohn's patients, many other conditions can arise because of your disease that require surgery to fix them. From experience, I know how embarrassing and uncomfortable fistulas can be, and medications alone may not always close these abnormal tunnels. Abscesses that become infected can lead to sepsis, and surgery can remove this tissue before it enters the bloodstream.

Drawbacks: First, it's important to note that nothing you do can cure you of your disease, even if you are a UC patient who has completely removed their colon. Surgery cannot make your body unlearn its inflammatory processes. You will still experience some version of your autoimmune disease, or even trigger a new autoimmune disease. When you surgically alter your body, in any way, what the surgeons do is irreversible. That is not to say that a failing j-pouch cannot be reversed back to an ileostomy, but that by cutting into you, surgeons irreparably create scar tissue. The way in which this forms is not controllable, and many may experience mechanical failure with regard to their surgery. For UC patients, several problems can arise after the surgery. For a number of unspecific years after the ileal-pouch anal anastomosis surgery (or, "take-down"), anywhere from 24% to 48% of patients will experience pouchitis, which is inflammation of the pouch that mimics colitis-like symptoms, while another 3% to 16% of

women who receive this surgery will develop pouch-vaginal fistulas that allow waste from the the pouch to secrete into the va-
ginal cavity (Hwang, 2008). In women who receive the surgery,
the rate of infertility is 38.6%, which is about four times greater
than that of the general population. A study into the quality of
life for patients after surgery found that fecal incontinence and
severe urgency were 7.3% and 8.5% respectively, after 60 months
post-op (Hueting et al. 2005). Where there is crossover or mis-
diagnosis following IPAA to Crohn's Disease, these rates are
shown to be significantly higher, and this surgery is not generally
recommended in Crohn's patients for these reasons. However,
bowel resection, surgery for fistulas, surgery for anorectal disease, and surgery for fissures are more likely surgeries. Unfortu-
nately, they often need to be performed multiple times in the
same patient, who will have recurrent issues with the same condition. Many of these surgeries have a relatively poor success rate
in themselves, owing to the unpredictability of inflammation
and active symptoms. I can tell you from experience, nothing is
worse than recovering from a surgery you know was a failure.

Side Effects: stenosis, stricture, infertility in women, bowel obstruction, short bowel, fecal incontinence, leakage, scarring,
weakened pelvic muscles, pouchitis, cuffitis, fistulas, dyspareu-
nia

It is important that you discuss the benefits and drawbacks of
any treatment with your doctor, because ultimately you will be
the one who needs to live with the consequences. However, I do
believe that some form of treatment needs to be in place for your
condition, no matter its severity, location, or impact on your
daily life. In UC, progress of the disease can be extremely gradual,
and often does not cause symptoms consistently enough that a
patient experiences a flare.

I also believe that there is no true diet out there that will help
you treat your condition, and I have therefore not listed diet as a

treatment option. While eliminating certain foods from your diet may help you prevent future triggers of relapse, or help you to manage your symptoms during a flare, no diet is a guarantee for all patients, and the foods that bother you may not bother others. For this reason, doctors do not usually tell patients to alter their diet as a part of their treatment. Certainly, doctors who treat you in a hospital may order NPO, liquids, or low-residue diets during your stay, but the only way to treat your chronic condition is with medication that will stop inflammation at its source.

One way you can do this holistically is to add the natural anti-inflammatory cannabidiol, or CBD, to your daily routine. In the next chapter, we'll cover why CBD works and for which symptoms. Do you have your app or the log of your symptoms handy? Then let's go over how CBD may address your symptoms or help keep you in remission longer.

Chapter Four

How CBD Can Help

CBD, or cannabidiol, is a product derived from hemp. It is a naturally occurring compound associated with the cannabis plant, but please do not be mistaken. This compound cannot get you high, a feeling that actually comes from THC, or tetrahydrocannabinol. In fact, most CBD products contain less than 0.3% of THC. CBD reacts differently with your endocannibinoid system (ECS), a system of receptors in your body which is "now known to regulate pain perception, gastrointestinal motility, immune function and many other systems in the body. Its receptors are located throughout the brain and body, including the entire gastrointestinal tract" (Weils, 2019).

CBD is generally legal as long as it contains .3% of THC, and can be ordered over the internet. It can come in many forms, which may suit you for different purposes. Though there is a lot of stigma attached to using it, it is a natural product that interacts with a system within our body that is meant for its consumption. In fact, studies done have found that there is "evidence that IBD patients had fewer endocannabinoids" (Dannels, 2018). This might indicate that patients who report relief after using cannabinoid products, of any strength, might be providing a balance in the CB1 and CB2 recepters, parts of the the ECS responsible for function in the brain and immune system, respectively (Nagarkatti et al. 2010). In fact, it has been posited that "The role of the ECS in gut homeostasis and its ability to modulate inflammatory responses demonstrate its part in preserving gastrointestinal function. Alterations of the ECS may predispose patients to pathologic disorders, including IBD" (Ahmed, 2016). Our lack of endocannibinoid production may intrinsically be connected to our body's CB2 receptors, which control our immune system and its response.

Knowing this, it may be possible to incorporate CBD into your daily life with moderately low risk of adverse side effects or habit-forming dependency. In fact, "only approximately 10% of cannabis users ever develop dependency, which is comparatively less than what is seen in tobacco, alcohol, cocaine, or heroin use" (Ahmed, 2016). Here are a few cases in which you must first determine that you are eligible to begin using CBD:

1. You are at least 25 years old, or if you are between the ages of 18 and 24, you have discussed your intent with a doctor

2. You do not take any blood thinners, such as Coumadin or Warfarin

3. You have recently tested negative for c. diff or have no symptoms of c. diff

4. Your condition has remained unchanged over the last 3 months, whether you are in remission or in a flare

5. You have not recently started a new diet or medication, especially immunomodulators or immunosuppressants

6. You do not have IBS, which you may have in addition to IBD. If you do, discuss CBD with your doctor, as no conclusive data supports any benefit of its use for IBS (Dannels, 2018)

7. You do not take any medications that caution against grapefruit, as CBD inhibits cytochrome p450 enzymes just like grapefruit does (Cadena, 2019)

Cbd For Mental Wellbeing

We've discussed already how stress is a major factor not only in shaping the conditions under which we first developed symptoms, but in the relapse of the disease during times where our symptoms flare. Whether this is a traumatic life event or a sustained period of stress from financial woes, the 2005 study in "Gut" states, "Both chronic stress and acute stress are associated with alterations in systemic immune and inflammatory function which may have relevance to the pathogenesis of IBD." During these times, our bodies respond by producing cortisol, an inflammatory hormone that is tied to the mechanism of all autoimmune diseases. In addition to this, the same study found that, "Acute psychological stress has effects on gastrointestinal motility, and water and ion secretion." These all play into the symptomatology of IBD, demonstrating how stress can trigger relapses by affecting the parts of us that are responsible for the way we feel during a flare. During periods of stress, our bodies also tolerate pain on a lower threshold than we normally do, making the onset of symptoms more acute and debilitating.

An article in The American Journal of Gastroenterology noted studies done into the rate of anxiety and depression among IBD patients, identifying that 19% of patients presented with anxiety and 9.2% presented with depression (Farraye et al. 2017). There was no difference in whether patients were in remission or relapse. The implications of this study on the IBD community is that, along with our rate of incidence for depression being higher than the average population's 6.7% (National Institute of Mental Health), nearly a quarter of all IBD patients live with chronic mental stress caused by these disorders. This means that in general, IBD patients are more susceptible to the effects of long-term stress on the body, which could play in important role in our likelihood of relapse. This was studied in 2004, showing an increased risk of relapse within eighteen months, depending on a patient's score on the Beck's Depression Inventory (Mawdsley, 2005). A study conducted in Boston area hospitals found that surgery for either Crohn's or UC increased these odds, citing the risk of depression or anxiety for Crohn's was 16% and 11% for ulcerative colitis within five years of their surgery (Ananthakrishnan et al. 2013).

In many studies performed to determine the impact of these disorders on remission success, several have found evidence that "in multivariate analysis that steroid intake and depression predicted worse disease outcomes" (Farraye et al. 2017) while others found that patients with depression who were not being treated for the disorder were significantly less likely to utilize their healthcare providers, even during a relapse. Therefore, it is imperative that IBD patients properly treat depression and anxiety, and discuss with their doctors any feelings they have of hopelessness, difficulty falling or staying asleep, inability to concentrate, racing thoughts, onset of strong negative thoughts, lack of desire to participate in previously enjoyable activities, and decreased feelings of satisfaction or sex drive.

In treating these symptoms, CBD is listed as having a possible benefit on mental disorders by the World Health Organization (WHO). By communicating with our ECS, it can send messages to our hippocampus that mimic its production of natural "feel good" molecules that promote the same feeling we get from relaxation, exercise, and sleeping well. "When CBD binds with your serotonin receptors, it can help reduce anxiety, pain, nausea, and sleep interruptions" (Zimmerman, 2019). In case studies done of social anxiety, researchers have found that instances of negative self-talk can decrease with use of CBD and that CBD can actually promote participation in social interaction (Bergamaschi et al. 2011). In fact, this can extend so far as to help overcome public speaking phobias.

In more serious disorders, CBD may be safer than other conventional drugs, which may inadvertently cause patients who also suffer from IBD to experience a relapse. A 2012 study cited by Psychology Today found that among patients suffering from psychosis, CBD was as beneficial in curbing episodes as antipsychotic drugs, with fewer side effects. Patients taking the CBD in the double blind experiment did not experience weight gain and increased appetite, sexual dysfunction, or hormonal imbalances. Many of these side effects could trigger a relapse in IBD patients, and CBD could more safely treat the symptoms of psychosis in order to avoid flares.

In the 1950's, Inflammatory Bowel Disease was classified as a psychosomatic disorder for a reason. It was clear, even then, that how we deal with stress and feelings of depression were largely tied to the onset and progression of Crohn's Disease and ulcerative colitis. In choosing to use CBD for your depression, anxiety, or other condition related to your mentality, think of how you want CBD to help you manage the symptoms that most affect your IBD. The goal is to break the vicious cycle that causes both conditions to continuously feed into one another, where suffering from constant pain and urgency to use the bathroom increases feelings of anxiety and depression, which then cause a worsening of these symptoms, only to trigger those feelings again. By adding CBD to your routine, you can reduce the feelings that feed your flare. If you have gone through surgery, you can use CBD to help promote your body's natural balance of endocannabinoids in your brain to better support the "feel good" sensation that your body requires in order to achieve homeostasis.

Urgency And Frequency

As previously discussed, the urge to go to the bathroom is the most common symptom reported by patients of both Crohn's Disease and ulcerative colitis. It may be connected to diarrhea that can often occur with both conditions, though sometimes it is simply a feeling with no real physiological need to pass stool. Frequency can be defined by The Mayo Clinic as more than 6 loose stools a day. The overactivity of the digestive tract's motility (movement) produces the feeling of tenesmus. Cannabidiol (CBD) has been shown to reduce motility of the gut, working as a natural antispasmodic. A study into the effects of CBD on the digestive tract stated, "In view of its low toxicity in humans, cannabidiol may represent a good candidate to normalize motility in patients with inflammatory bowel disease" (Capasso et al. 2008).

Again, this all ties to how our CB1 and CB2 receptors interpret our brain's messages. The signals produced in these receptors interact with the endocannibinoid system to provide the brain and immune system "status reports" of the body that can activate an immune response, or calm it. "Activation of these receptors may help reduce intestinal transit time and reduce colon propulsion," one study claims (Kafil et al. 2018).

If you do want to use CBD to cut down on the number of bathroom trips you make or the constant pressure to go caused by the inflammation in your digestive tract, you want to consider how its antispasmodic properties may decrease the hyper motility (constant movement) of your gut. In the next chapter, we'll discuss forms of CBD that do this best and how to measure your need for it in this capacity.

Pain

Pain is a difficult symptom to live with when relief does not seem possible. Whether abdominal cramping or soreness from using the bathroom repeatedly, the arthritic pains of inflammation in your joints or the discomfort of constipation and hemorrhoids, Inflammatory Bowel Disease can be very painful. This is because the inflammation running rampant through a patient's digestive tract causes pain as food passes through it, either as the food scrapes areas of tender and exposed tissue, or as the muscles contract repeatedly in irritation. However, CBD has antispasmodic properties. An article on the subject claims,

"CBD will also relax the contractions of intestinal muscles, which usually lead to abdominal pain" (Dannels, 2018). Not only can it help with the cramping you feel as these muscles contract, but CBD naturally binds to a pain receptor responsible for pain, essentially blocking it from receiving pain signals (Zimmerman, 2019).

When patients experience relapse of their disease, and how long that lasts, has a significant impact on their toleration of pain. The vicious cycle between stress and symptoms needs to be broken. In this regard, CBD has a double purpose. By controlling the stress placed on the body with CBD it is possible to interrupt your body's production of cortisol, an inflammatory hormone, as well as to curb the immune response of attacking T-cells as it binds with the CB2 receptors that are responsible for your body's immune response. In fact, "CB2 receptor activation may lead to T-cell apoptosis, decreased T-cell proliferation in colitis, decreased recruitment of leukocytes to the inflamed colon, and may also help reduce the release of cytokines" (Kafil et al. 2018). The 2005 study in "Gut" stated, "laboratory research has indicated a variety of mechanisms by which stress can affect both the systemic and gastrointestinal immune and inflammatory responses" (Mawdsley, 2005). By interrupting the mechanisms controlled by both CB1 and CB2 receptors, the systemic inflammation that causes pain might be affected. However, many studies have found that while patients with Crohn's might feel a relief of symptoms, CBD by itself does not actually reduce inflammation in the gut (Naftali et al. 2017). In UC, similar results have found that though it does not reduce inflammation on its own, it has powerful effects on the inflammation of the colon when administered as a hybrid (Pagano et al. 2016) and can help some patients achieve clinical remission where conventional methods fail (Ahmed, 2016).

As surgery is likely for about a half of Crohn's patients, and a quarter of UC patients (keeping in mind that statistics for surgery past the thirty year mark are scarce), even drastic measures to alleviate the debilitation of these conditions does not necessarily eradicate pain. Thus, "Patients with a history of abdominal surgery, chronic analgesic use, CAM use, and a lower Short Inflammatory Bowel Disease Questionnaire score were more likely to use cannabis for symptom relief" (Ahmed, 2016). This more than matches current research on IBD patients, finding that over half already use cannabis in one form or another, either for acute or chronic symptoms (Irving et al. 2015). Especially in Crohn's patients, it may also be able to help avoid surgery. An Israeli study of 30 patients found that within a nine year period, 15 needed surgery at least once. In the following three years that the patients used cannabis, only 2 required surgery (Naftali et al. 2011).

When our bodies are stressed by either external forces or the inflammation affecting our guts, our threshold for pain is lowered as a survival instinct in our CB1 receptors, which we've previously discussed is tied to the endocannibinoid system, and then spreads throughout the nervous system, peripheral tissues and gastrointestinal system. In the central nervous system, according to one study that sought to utilize cannabinoids for UC, "CB1 receptors are associated with effects such as reduction in pain and nausea" (Kafil, 2018). By introducing a "supplement" of CBD into your system, you can effectively shut off your CB1 response to a flare, thereby controlling your pain threshold.

However, the CB2 receptor does not control the root of the pain, which is a symptom of the inflammation throughout the affected tissue in the mucosa of the digestive system. After studying the effect of cannabis for pain management the 2008 study in The British Journal of Pharmacology stated, "Another possible target of the CBD action is the cannabinoid CB2 receptor. In the gut, this receptor has been found to be expressed by inflammatory/immune cells and also identified on epithelial cells and neurons" (Capasso et al. 2008). By controlling the amount of inflammation likely to occur at its source, the hope is that it will curb the symptoms and progression of the disease. Another study took a similar approach to this position in its research into the control of moderate to severe UC, with the intent to help patients achieve clinical remission. The study claimed, "CB2 receptor activation may lead to T-cell apoptosis, decreased T-cell proliferation in colitis, decreased recruitment of leukocytes to the inflamed colon, and may also help reduce the release of cytokines" (Kafil et al. 2018). However, other resources have found that by itself, CBD cannot reduce inflammation in patients with Crohn's Disease, only curb symptoms (Zimmerman, 2019). It can, however, provide relief of symptoms, especially when conventional drugs cannot fully control symptoms, and should be studied further for use as a holistic therapy (Ahmed, 2016).

This is a more natural, less risky way of addressing how your body perceives pain than narcotics (which are habit-forming and dangerous for long-term use), NSAIDS (which are not recommended in IBD patients due to their potential to worsen inflammation and cause bleeding), or acetaminophen (which puts strain on your liver and may interfere with other medications and alcohol). Many studies have taken note of patients' ability to taper off of corticosteroids while using CBD and other cannabis products and the high success rates of symptom improvement (Naftali et al. 2013). In some cases, these success rates were higher than they were with certain conventional drug therapies (Lal, 2011).

Nausea And Vomiting

Nausea and vomiting are common with IBD, more so as the severity of the disease progresses. As a result, patients with IBD are susceptible to weight loss, vitamin deficiency, and loss of water retention. Doctors may prescribe common anti-emetic drugs like Zofran or Tramadol to counteract these symptoms, but their common side effects might be just as detrimental to a patient in an active flare. Using these medications daily may cause dizziness, diarrhea, weakness, and feelings of tiredness, and might exacerbate these symptoms if already present.

For some patients who do not tolerate these medications well, or for patients who infrequently experience nausea but do not have a prescription, CBD might be a better alternative. "Various CBD formulations have been tested in pre-clinical studies to have diverse medicinal properties, such as anti-nausea, anti-emetic, anti-tumor, anti-inflammatory, anti-depressant, anti-psychotic, and anti-anxiolytic" claims one article (Taylor & Sauls, 2019). This may also help patients who suffer nausea even if currently medicated for their condition who do not see an improvement with this symptom, or find that their medication increases these feelings. Studies into using CBD concomitantly with certain 5-ASA drugs actually increased the effectiveness of the medication, particularly in reducing the inflammation that affects the nervous system's mode of transport between the gut and amygdala, which helps to process sensory information (Irving et al. 2018).

CBD affects nausea and vomiting as it interacts with the CB1 receptors associated with the ECS, which is most centrally located in the central nervous system. The receptors respond through "physiological and pathophysiological actions in the gastrointestinal tract (e.g., peristalsis, secretion, gastric emptying, emesis, satiety, immunomodulation/inflammation and pain)" (Irving et al. 2018). Cannabinoids have been studied for their effect on appetite and emesis since the 1980's, and multiple studies have concluded that they are at least as effective as typical anti-emetics with few side effects, even in the few studies that have been done involving children (Parker et al. 2011). For those patients with mild to moderate IBD, who do not experience full remission using 5-ASA's a combination therapy with CBD might improve its success rather than move to more invasive drug therapies, which often increase the feelings of emesis.

Next Steps

Choosing to use CBD for symptom relief may be an important step for you in controlling how you feel, whether you are in remission or relapse, and the use of it may very well increase your quality of life. Your goal now should be zeroing in on a symptom that you feel impacts your ability to enjoy your life. It could be more than one. If you've really taken the time to record your symptoms and track their effect on your daily life over the course of at least a few days, you're ready to dive in to purchasing products that will best support your intent. So let's make sure you know what you are looking for:

<u>Prevalence and Frequency of Symptoms:</u> How and when you take medications depends on how you perceive their ability to help you. You don't wake up and take Tylenol each morning as a part of your routine as a rule, because our use of over the counter pain medications is usually a response to pain we have at the time we take it. We don't only take our prescribed medications on the days we have symptoms because we know that its benefit to maintenance in remission depends on its consistency in our routine. Just like with any other things you use to treat your illness, CBD should be taken a certain way. It's up to you to decide if you want to use it proactively or reactively. So decide what your approach should begin with. Ask yourself a few questions to help you decide if you want to use CBD proactively or reactively:

1) Do I experience my symptoms every day, or are my symptoms infrequent?

2) Are my symptoms chronic or acute, meaning I either experience them all the time for long periods of time or suddenly out of the blue?

3) How do I think I can manage a new supplement in my schedule?

Timing: Thinking about your routine and your symptoms, you might be able to make a decision about how you want to use CBD based on time-related data that might indicate that you want to use CBD proactively to avoid the onset of certain symptoms. Perhaps you've noticed that increased urgency or frequency correlates to meals or to a certain caloric intake. Or that it's hard to fall asleep because of stomach cramping. If you have been documenting your symptoms, look them over for trends in the timing or overall part of the day where they are worse. Next, review a few things:

1) Are your symptoms more frequent during a certain segment of the day, or relatively constant?

2) When you do have symptoms, does something consistently precede them, like a workout or a meal?

3) Does something make them worse, like traveling or working?

Mentality: Though it may not be because of an underlying mental disorder, your mood and stress level can exacerbate your symptoms, or even, as we've gone over with pain threshold, your ability to tolerate your symptoms. Therefore, expecting that you will not feel necessarily positive or happy as you experience symptoms can help you plan for your mentality as a part of your overall wellness plan. CBD might, again, be a proactive choice you make at the earliest onset of symptoms, or that you use before a particularly stressful event in your day. Planning for CBD use as an integral part of your mental health can help you break the cycle of pain and stress, so let's consider:

1) Would you benefit from anxiety control, particularly if you are in a flare or get anxious about going places where you might not have a bathroom?

2) Does your mood or your stress level affect your symptoms, either the onset of them or the level of their severity?

3) Do you often feel the need to go to the bathroom just by worrying about it, e.g. when stuck in traffic or in the middle of teaching a lesson?

You deserve to feel symptom and stress-free. CBD might help you achieve one or both of these outcomes with careful planning and control of the factors that may normally affect you. If you do plan to use CBD and you're ready to buy some products that will be the most use for your particular symptoms, it's important to know what products fit you best. In the next chapter, we'll look at the various methods of use and how each is different for what you want CBD to do. Depending on whether you want to use CBD every day proactively, or only for certain symptoms as they arise, the method of use is critical to your success.

Chapter Five

Finding Products That
Are Right For You

CBD, or cannabidiol, is a non-psychoactive derivative of the hemp plant, along with 112 other cannibinoids, including THC. Though CBD does not get you high, and is perfectly legal to order online or in certain CBD shops as an oil, CBD does usually contain trace amounts of THC, though it can be as little as 0.3% (Weil, 2019). When choosing CBD products, your optimal purchase will be a combination of the best method of delivery for your symptoms and convenience for your life, though it is also important for consumers to be cost effective. Most of all, a balance of optimal bioavailability for your specific symptoms. Bioavailability will be discussed often moving forward. By definition, "Bioavailability is the amount of CBD that actually stays in the system to perform its work" (Nede, 2018).

Many people who take it worry that it could show up in a drug test. Though it is possible if you choose a Full Spectrum product that enters your bloodstream, it should not be a concern for you as long as you are using CBD that has had THC removed. This comes in two forms: CBD Isolate and Broad Spectrum. I recommend using Broad Spectrum products because it contains several other cannabinoids as well besides just CBD, which can give you the "entourage effect," which simply means you get more of a benefit from multiple cannabinoids than you do from only one, which has been noted to be particularly effective in controlling inflammation (Nagarkatti et al. 2010). These will also test negative in drug screenings, as the THC has been stripped from the extract that produces Broad Spectrum.

It can be taken in a variety of ways, and the different methods for delivery into your body can have different effects. In all cases, the actual component is added to an essential oil, or fatty oil such as coconut, to act as a vehicle for its delivery to your system. There are a few things you might want to think about when buying products, and some of them do not relate in any way to your symptoms. Since you've probably already decided whether you want to focus on chronic or acute symptoms for now, let's review a few other questions you need answer:

1) How much money are you willing to spend on products?
2) Where and when do you plan to use CBD?
3) What preferences do you have? Is there a method that is unappealing?
4) How much of an effect are you looking for from your products?

Cost: As we go through products, I'll make sure to give you estimates for what you can expect to spend. Typically, cost varies by strength and type of product. For example, you can spend a lot or a little on some products that have a low, medium, or high potency option, but certain methods of delivery into your system will be more expensive than others in general. If you are not looking to spend a lot, you may have fewer options that suit your needs. However, there will certainly be options for your budget regardless. Think about this: what do you ideally want to spend a month? It might end up being very much or very little, depending on if you want to use CBD daily or only once in a while, as well as if you have a particular preference. Not only can you save by using low potency or choosing not to use CBD every day, but you can also save money by choosing appropriate products for your symptoms, which will ensure that you don't waste the bioavailability of your CBD needlessly.

Method of Delivery: I'll spend most of the chapter diving into the differences between methods of delivery, but it's important that you get an idea of how CBD products can be divided between acute and chronic use now. Based on how you want to use CBD to treat symptoms either as they happen acutely or daily as a supplement to treat chronic symptoms, or even proactively to keep them at bay, you may want to review your options within that category and think about one or two you would prefer.

Acute- inhalation, sublingual, rectal

Chronic- oral, edible, topical

Convenience: It might be worth taking a moment to envision how you'll use CBD. I can tell you from experience that it can be difficult to use CBD right away for acute symptoms if you're taking an L Train to Brooklyn if all you've got on you is a vape pen, even if it would earn you a gajillion hipster points. So, especially if you sometimes have acute symptoms while out in public, be mindful that some forms of CBD are easier than others to tote around. If you're at home with kids, and worried they might eat your CBD cookies, maybe a capsule is less enticing. Whatever you pick, you want it to work for your lifestyle and your condition.

Potency: As you begin buying products, you'll notice that the price goes up with the potency of the CBD. This can be tricky, because you'll be tempted to get the most concentrated amount for the best price. However, research suggests beginning slow. This is because you may end up overpaying for results you could have achieved at a lower dose, and at high doses, you may build up a tolerance that you can't sustain long-term (Greenhut, 2019). No one wants to spend money needlessly, so instead of going straight for the "Big Kahuna" (a 1,000 or 5,000 mg) product, start with maybe 100 mg to 150 mg. Naftali and colleagues prescribed a potency of 115 mg in their controlled study (2013). This will also give you room to scale up to a higher potency if you think you could experience even better results. At the higher potencies, "you don't have much room to increase your dosage or experiment to see what helps you best" claims Greenhut, of GreenPath

Science. As there are yet few studies that have measured the success of CBD at varying potency levels, you will have to do some experimentation yourself to find a dosage that works the way you need it to.

<u>Product Type:</u> As much as all CBD products contain CBD, it wouldn't be fair to assume that all products have the same effect on you. Therefore, you need to consider what kind of effect on you you're looking for CBD to have. I have terrible arthritis in my hands at times, so do I really expect a capsule to specifically target that pain once I ingest it? It could help, but it's not a direct method of delivery. I'd have much better results from a topical cream (and I've got a wonderful lavender cream I discovered in Pike Place Market that I'm dying to tell you about).

The same can be said for a Crohn's patient versus a UC patient, believe it or not. Or even a J-poucher or Ostomate! Think about it. If our disease is located on in our rectum right now, or you've had the surgery but experience cuffitis or fissures, do you really want to wait for an edible or capsule to travel all the way through you? By the time it does, you might get the benefit of less than 20% of the product's bioavailability (Nede, 2018). A suppository, the other hand, is much more likely to absorb straight into the inflamed tissue and ease the body's production of that inflammation as the suppository slowly dissolves. Be purposeful in choosing the product that actually addresses your needs so you can not only experience the best possible benefit from CBD, but also get the most out of your money at the same time.

Inhalation

<u>Bioavailability:</u> up to 50%
<u>Time to full effect:</u> about 30 minutes
<u>Price Range:</u> Vape pen or kit can be anywhere from $15 to $50 (the

pens being cheaper), the cartridges and oils you add to these to burn into smoke can be anywhere from about $30-$600; CBD joints can be $15-$40 depending on how many joints come together

By smoking or vaping CBD, you can experience its effects within seconds. It is best for acute symptoms like severe stomach cramping, diarrhea at least three times in an hour, or symptoms that make it hard to perform basic tasks. Vaping or smoking delivers the compound directly into your system either by being brought into the lungs where it will mix with oxygen and be carried around your body, or by holding the smoke in your mouth for a few second where it will be absorbed by the capillaries under your tongue. Holding it in your mouth increases the product's bioavailability and removes some of the risk that comes with the effects of smoking.

The biggest advantages to using inhalation as your method of delivery is that it is the quickest and most bioavailable, meaning that no matter your symptoms, you know that using this product will be the most cost-effective and convenient, depending on how much you need it. Indeed, a pen is small and compact and can be as a cheap as fifteen dollars. It's very inconspicuous and produces very little smoke. It can be flavored to cover the taste of the hemp. If you are at home and need something quickly to control an acute attack of symptoms, it's most likely to be useful on short notice without needing to wait long for its effects to kick in.

If you are using a CBD joint, it may be less possible to measure how much you consume from a couple of puffs. Additionally, these are less likely to be flavored and may draw unwanted attention in public, as they will have a hemp odor that is similar to THC. They're also harder to save, so if you begin to smoke one and feel better, you might be tempted to finish the whole joint. In this way, it might not be as cost effective. It also carries many of the same risks as smoking a regular cigarette, just like using a vaporizer. Patients are more likely to have bronchial infections if they smoke CBD (Ahmed, 2016). However, a study in the Harm Reduction Journal states that, "Components of cannabis smoke minimize some carcinogenic pathways whereas tobacco smoke enhances some" (2005). Therefore, smoking CBD is not linked to increased risk of cancer. However, be careful not to overheat your vaporizer because doing so can convert the liquid into harmful benzenes, found one research article (2017). Expect the effects to be short-lived; like our view of steroids, inhalation is a "quick fix" for acute symptoms.

Product Suggestions:

CBDfx- This is an online site for CBD products of all kinds, rated the best CBD vape pen in 2020 by Vaping360. It offers a vaporizer kit for as little a $39.99. They also sell disposable pens for about $15, which come in a lot of different flavors. They offer broad spectrum products and you can even view the lab reports for each product to see exactly what it contains and how much. They're disposable, so you simply order another when you've used it up.

Purekana- These products are all pure CBD, and again, offer lab reports for you to view. What I love about these products is that they've already done the math; they can estimate what I'm getting out of a serving and take bioavailability into consideration. It can even tell you the average number of servings you get out of it! Each product comes with suggestions for use, to maximize the product's benefits. Surprisingly, different strains or added ingredients affect you differently.

Secret Nature- This site has a wide range of products that include both broad spectrum and full spectrum. Though navigating the products for pure CBD is harder with this mixture of THC-free or hybrid blends, a well-informed consumer can find practically anything they could need here, from CBD flower to rare cannabinoid extracts. They have a range of products that includes pre-rolls (joints), vaporizers, and bundles that allow you to roll your own.

Sublingual Tincture

<u>Bioavailability:</u> 20-30%
<u>Time to full effect:</u> 30-60 minutes
<u>Price Range:</u> About $15 (125 mg) to $400 (5,000 mg)

CBD oils are bottled and sold with droppers in the lid so that you can draw out measured amounts of the compound and then squeeze the contents out under your tongue. You hold the liquid there for up to 90 seconds as it absorbs slowly through the capillaries there in the same manner as it does when you vape the smoke of CBD and hold it in your mouth. The idea in doing this is that you avoid introducing CBD to your liver, which will metabolize the product faster than your body can process its effects on you. This is why, even though you can add a dropper of the liquid to a favorite beverage, I do not recommend that you do this. This essentially eliminates half of the bioavailability of the CBD.

Taking CBD sublingually has a lot of advantages. For one, it's extremely easy to use, as most droppers come with measurements along the side, if you're trying out varying amounts to find your optimal level. It doesn't generally have a strong taste, and the essential oil that binds it for optimal delivery can be flavored with some of your favorite aromas. Personally, lavender is my favorite scent, and I can order it on Amazon from Select Hemp! It's less noticeable in public than a vape or joint, and much more controlled than smoking can be if you measure the amount and count the same number of seconds each time. For patients with trouble swallowing or breathing deeply, this will not be necessary when using a tincture.

It isn't everyone's cup of tea, however. For people with nausea, holding a liquid with a slightly "off" taste in your mouth might increase the sensation of needing to vomit (Dannels, 2018). For others who do not like the taste, I would recommend trying a tincture made with a flavored essential oil rather than hide the dropper full of liquid in a drink, which as I've said, lowers the product's bioavailability. You cand also add your own essential oil to it to "water down" the taste and increase bioavailability. The tincture is also not the most convenient of methods if out in public or traveling, as you need to handle the bottle and the dropper without the jostle of public transit. In general I don't suggest traveling with CBD unless you've researched ahead of time that it is permitted for flying and kept it in a checked bag.

<u>Product Suggestions:</u>

cbdMD- This online retailer sells one of the top rated CBD tinctures of 2020, according to CBDoilusers.com. The site offers flavors on each of its products and provides not only the ingredients and lab results you should come to demand from your retailer, but also a 60-day money back guarantee. The brand features fully vegan products, and carries extremely high potencies.

Hemp Bombs- Vaping360 rated this retailer its top pick for tinctures in 2020. The tinctures come in six awesome flavors (try the watermelon) and scales its prices incredibly well. Expect to pay $15 for every 125 mg a product contains. In case you wanted even more information on the endocannibinoid system (ECS), their homepage is very informative, even providing a diagram of the system on a human body for you to see.

NanocraftCBD- This site specializes in high potency formulas as well, but has an added twist I haven't come across anywhere else. They've developed formulas for use either during the day or at night, as well as their high potency Gold Series. The day formula is infused with B-12 and caffeine, while the night formula is infused with the scent of lavender and a touch of melatonin. You can save money by using the "subscribe and save" option, just as you would on Amazon.

Suppositories

<u>Bioavailability:</u> 80%-90%
<u>Time to full effect:</u> about 10 minutes
<u>Price Range:</u> About $20-$80 per 7 suppositories, 8, or 10 suppositories

Suppositories are something many IBD patients use already to control their symptoms, so it should not come as a surprise that big brand companies have figured out there's a high demand for rectal CBD use. In fact the content director of one of my favorite brands, Foria, describes the use of CBD "by imagining them as powerful topicals – except they are applied internally." There are three main arteries in the tush that can deliver the product into your bloodstream, and only one of these leads to the liver. Because of this, the suppository acts fast and retains almost all of its bioavailability.

It is certainly the most effective method of delivery, and can almost instantly relieve symptoms of tenesmus, burning, pressure, discomfort, or pain to a commonly affected area of disease activity for many patients. J-pouchers and patients with distal proctitis or pancolitis may find that they help relieve the urgency to go to the bathroom during the night if taken before bed. This is also a great method if you have trouble taking CBD orally. The effects of a suppository also last much longer than inhalation or tinctures, staying in your system for up to six hours.

Suppositories might not be the most convenient way to use CBD when you're out publicly, though they're great for traveling. They're also more expensive when you look at how many uses you get out of a box. Some come with 7, 8, or 10 to a box, but each is meant for a single use. This is quite a lot to spend if you intend to use them daily, as a box of 10 can go for $50. However, for those who want to use them only for acute symptoms, such as if they eat something that doesn't agree with them, or for temporary issues such as fissure or hemorrhoids, it might be more efficient than other methods of delivery.

Product Suggestions:

Foria- This is one of the top rated CBD suppository retailers of 2020, as rated by cbdbreaker.com. They have a higher potency than other brands offer for their suppositories, though this makes them a little more expensive. They're mainly marketed towards inflammation, but the site also offers suggestions for use for those interested in controlling various types of pain.

CBD Living- Not only is this the #1 rated seller for CBD suppositories, by several organizations, but they're a great buy for beginners, as their potency is rather mild. These do contain THC, but here's the fun bit: suppositories are much less likely than other methods to deliver the THC into your system because it isn't processed by your liver. So it doesn't show up in a drug test! This company sells suppositories in a pack of 10 for $50. Definitely an affordable option for beginners.

Palmetto Harmony- This company sells a pack of 7 suppositories for $20, which is great for beginners who aren't sure they want to invest a lot of money right away. The product is full spectrum so it does have THC, but again, should not be a problem if you're looking to avoid its psychoactive effects. The terpenes in this product help you get that "entourage effect" of benefits from multiple cannabinoids at once.

Capsules

Bioavailability: 6-10%

<u>Time to full effect:</u> About 2 hours
<u>Price Range:</u> About $50-100 for a 30 day supply

Capsules can be taken orally containing a broad range of ingredients, so it's important to pay attention to what fat or oil the CBD is paired with to make sure you get the most out of the product's bioavailability. In particular, MCT oil, or Medium Chain Triglycerides, is an important oil that is usually combined with the compound. Check the products ahead of time for this ingredient, and if it is not present, look for the retailer's ingredient list for other oils that will guarantee the product binds properly during transit through your digestive system. You can take them a few hours before bed to get a better night's sleep, or after a long day's work.

Capsules are easy for most of us to incorporate into our regimens because we probably already take pills. They're also convenient for taking in public or for traveling with. They are best used for systemic pain or mental disorders, as they enter the bloodstream after transit through the digestive tract and are delivered throughout the body. Since the capsules are already measured, it's a safe bet that you get the same dose every time. Unlike tinctures and inhalation, where you might absorb different amounts depending on your own actions, capsules are digested uniformly. They're also great for beginners who shy away from products with a distinct hemp taste, as they are completely tasteless.

If you have problems taking pills, this method may not be for you. It's also not for those who have no corresponding pill regimen with the time of day. If you are already prescribed a medication with a sedative effect, like narcotics, SSRI's, MAOI's, or antihistamines, talk to your doctor first before thinking of using ingestion as your method of CBD intake, as ingesting CBD and other medications that cause sleepiness together can cause the additive effect, "meaning they can increase the effects of the medication" (Cadena, 2019). It is also recommended that you speak to a doctor if you take certain epilepsy medications or undergo chemotherapy, as CBD can inhibit these drugs' full effect on you. If your other medications contraindicate CBD, I recommend methods other than ingestion for your CBD.

<u>Product Suggestions:</u>

Lazarus Naturals- This brand is completely vegan and non-GMO that uses coconut oil as its fat of choice for delivery to your system. If you're not ready to invest a lot of money until you're sure capsules are for you, Lazarus gives you a choice of capsules as low as 10 to a bottle for $15. The brand has CBD isolate and full spectrum choices and proudly describes its extraction process for costumers to read.

CBDistillery- Top Choice Reviews and Vaping360 rate this brand as one of the best, and its capsules are no exception. The company has both full spectrum and broad spectrum choices, so no matter your choice you can be assured you'll get the "entourage effect" of multiple cannabinoids. A 30-day supply sells for $60-$65, so be sure you are ready for the investment when you visit this site.

Joy Organics- This brand has the #1 rated capsule of 2020 according to Top Choice Reviews, with very good reason. Not only does the brand use nano emulsion to guarantee 200% bioavailability of the product, but it also uses that special MCT oil to help deliver the CBD to your system, working against your stomach acid to preserve the integrity of the compound. The brand is more expensive than others for a 30-day supply ($39.95 for 10 mg, $74.95 for 25mg), but there are more options for your wellbeing if you're willing to pay a little more. The brand also sells a capsuled infused with melatonin for sleep, and another infused with curcumin for inflammation. Both are priced at $89.95.

Edibles

<u>Bioavailability:</u> 13-19%
<u>Time to full effect:</u> About 2 hours
<u>Price Range:</u> As low as $6-$10 for single use edible, up to $50 for a 30 count of gummies (300 mg)

Edible products range from candies or chocolate to tea or coffee, all infused with the beneficial effects of CBD. Like capsules, the gummies are already measured with a specific potency in mind. These can be taken every day, like a capsule or suppository, or used only as needed, like vaping. For IBD patients who suffer from anxiety in public situations or who tend to worry about needing bathrooms when traveling abroad or to a new place. I ate a particularly potent chewable the moment my tour guide told us it would take us over an hour to travel between Pisa and Florence on a vacation I took with my husband and his family. I'd already spend at least five euros using a McDonald's bathroom in Pisa and I knew we wouldn't be stopping.

Edibles are a fun way to explore products that easily fit your daily routine, while also providing you with your favorite treat. Since they can be sold in monthly supplies, bundles, or singles, they're a versatile option for beginners who want to take some time exploring options. They can also be infused into coffee, tea, drink powder, candy, chocolate, dried fruit, cookies, and more. This makes them a delicious alternative to other methods of delivery, and most brands are vegan and GMO-free. Brands also offer varieties that have added bonuses for your health, like vitamins or supplements you may already use. They're one of the best options for cost and convenience, so if you haven't ever tried CBD before, this might be where you want to start. They are also the most effective method for those trying to gain weight, battling nausea, or overcoming an eating disorder (Nede, 2018).

Always remember to take into account that most of the bioavailability of ingested CBD products is lost on its way through your digestive tract, and you can increase bioavailability by eating something oily right before or right after ingesting it. Make sure you check the ingredients of each product before selecting your choice to check that some sort of fat is included in the design. For this reason, I suggest staying away from teas, coffees, shot boosters, and drink powders unless you plan to use these in conjunction with another method. They often contain sugars, which will cause the product to move faster through you before it can be absorbed, and may aggravate some IBD symptoms or contraindicate certain diets that eliminate sugars. Chocolate and candies contain natural fats that make it a better option, and by holding the treat in your mouth or thoroughly chewing, you can increase its bioavailability.

Product Suggestions:

Green Roads- This retailer has won the Cannabis Business Awards for 2018 and 2019, and was a top seller in 2020 as well. For beginners, this is the best site to visit for single-use products, like their Sleepy Z's. They also have a line of coffees and teas that have been infused with CBD. Enjoy their blend of chamomile before bed for a great night's rest. Each product comes with lab reports and recommendations for use, so it is informative for new customers who might want common questions answered. Since the products are all very cheap for single or double use, you can stock up on a variety before deciding on a favorite.

Savage CBD- This retailer has a little bit of everything, including wellness shots 3-packs for $19.99. They sell high potency gummies in packs of 6, perfect if you're new to edibles or if you suffer acute symptoms only once in a while. The retailer offers other fun options like pink lemonade drink powder and a bundle of its edible products for $50. It's been rated one of the top edibles sellers by Leafreport, and sells both CBD isolate and full spectrum products.

Verma Farms- This brand doesn't just offer gummies like a lot of brands do, but you can also get CBD dried fruit. All edibles come in low and high potency forms, so you can scale your dose up or down. The gummies are made with real fruit flavor, so you know you're getting the added bonus of those vitamins when you eat them. If you know you love these, buy them in a bundle to make your purchase more cost effective.

Topical

<u>Bioavailability:</u> N/A
<u>Time to full effect:</u> Within 20 minutes
<u>Price Range:</u> As low as $6-$8, as much as $150 for a kit

Topical CBD methods of delivery come in a wide range, the most versatile by far of all method types. They can come as lip balms, ointments, creams, roll-on sticks, salves, lotions, bath bombs, serum, sun screen, face masks, sprays, shampoos, and body wash. Essentially, topical CBD methods enter the first three layers of your skin, where "there are more CB2 and TRPV1 receptors in your skin and periphery system than CB1 receptors," meaning that your body interacts with the CBD in the receptors responsible for your inflammatory response (Mannino, 2019). For patients who suffer from arthritis in the joints, a common symptom of any autoimmune disease, this product can help relieve the affect joints when applied directly to the area. It goes to work pretty quickly to calm these receptors. Additionally, a CBD serum, lotion, cream, or salve can be applied to surgical scars and has the same effect on it that a scar eraser would, with the added bonus that you are allowing the CBD to aid the pain receptors in those areas.

Topical CBD methods can be used in any number of ways to relieve aching, soreness, arthritis, dryness, nerve pain, and surgical scarring however you wish to use them. They go to work fast, so you can expect relief soon after application. Small bottles or jars can be carried at east when you're traveling, and best of all, the compound will never enter your bloodstream. This means you can use THC-infused products without fear of mood altering or false positive drug tests. It also means that you can use the product at any time without a sedative effect. The effects on your pain can last up to 4 hours, which makes it a more direct and equally effective option than OTC pain relievers for arthritic pains. I discovered a glorious lavender scented balm at "All Things Lavender" in the Pike Place Market while visiting Seattle in 2019. It's just behind the fish mongers, and you can visit their shop online at https://www.allthingslavenderseattle.com/ for more information on how to purchase their CBD products. I rub some into my knuckles and feel so relieved.

Topical CBD products will not control most IBD symptoms because they will not interact with the CB1 receptors to induce serotonin production or signal homeostasis to the brain. If you are looking for help controlling anxiety or depression, this method will not affect your mood in any way. Using it daily will not help you stay in or remission or help you out of a flare, so limit your expectations of a topical product. They are often confused with transdermal suppositories, but remember that suppositories enter your bloodstream via any of the three major arteries there. A topical treatment affects only the part of the skin where it is applied, and therefore does not travel systemically. It's also impossible to measure the effectiveness of a product's bio-availability over another simply by strength, so do not be fooled by high potency items. Instead, look for menthol, LCT (long-chain triglyceride), MCT, and other natural oils.

Product Suggestions:

CBD Medic- You might have heard of the brand because Rob Gronkowski endorses their products, and in fact it's a well-known name in football. This site is dedicated to pain relief and using natural ingredients that are hypoallergenic and cruelty-free. The site has products for skincare as well. Each product has suggestions for application, and many are designed for specific join pain. Their ointments go for about $39.99 a bottle, and they also sell serums, sticks, sprays, cleansers, and creams.

Charlotte's Web- If you're new to topical treatments and want to try cheaper options first, this retailer sells roll-ons, gels, creams, and balms for as little as $14.99. They're vegan and designed for sensitive skin, as well as cruelty-free. They offer Subscribe and Save options once you know you love the product for extra savings.

Discover CBD- This site has more variety than the other two and is cruelty-free. You can try out single-use products like their bath bombs or patches for as little as $8-$9 or invest in bundles of lip balms and creams. Planning to travel? They sell travel sizes. The website offers free shipping on all orders thatpwithin the U.S.

Conclusion

Now that you've read about each method of delivery, and you've compared either your own research or my suggestions to each point of consideration in preparing to make your purposes, you're ready to start ordering products that appeal to you. I'll include a few resources at the end of this book that you can reference to find out your state's current views on cannabis, though it should be noted that all 50 states currently recognize CBD as a legal substance. However, certain restrictions might be placed on shipping CBD products over state lines in some places. I'll also include helpful apps or websites you might want to visit to find CBD stores or dispensaries in your area, as well as products or brands I have not explicitly mentioned.

CBD cannot cure you of your Inflammatory Bowel Disease, and it should not be used as an alternative to medications your doctor may have prescribed. Rather, CBD should be treated as a wellness supplement that you use to further benefit your body in a holistic way. If the goal is to maintain remission for as long as possible and potentially avoid surgery, CBD is a safe and low-risk way to explore a change in your lifestyle that could provide a multitude of benefits.

Remember that the best product for you will not be the same for everyone with Inflammatory Bowel Disease, as both Crohn's and UC are highly individualistic in nature. Careful trial and error may take time and patience, so don't become discouraged if you do not notice any benefit after only a week of consistent use. You didn't see immediate results with your maintenance medications, right? Try making any one of the following adjustments, only attempting one at a time for definitive results:

Potency- Adjust by 25 mg or 50 mg
Method of Delivery- Adjust to another pertinent method for either acute or chronic symptoms
Schedule- If no discernible change is noted while trying to fall asleep, for example, try adjusting the time at which you take it by a half hour the next night and keep doing this until a change is noted

Attempt the adjustment for at least a week before trying again with either the same adjustment type or a different one. Keeping notes of your CBD dosage and schedule will help you make more educated changes, which will ultimately cost you less money. Also make sure that as you use products, you follow product suggestions and recommendations for use.

It is important to talk to your doctor about anything you supplement, so being open about your CBD and your purpose for its use will help your doctor make informed decisions about other medications you take for your condition, as well as any other supplements or medications you take. Speak with your doctor at follow-up visits about how it has helped you, and specifically with which symptoms you notice this. If you want to attempt a diet to help you eliminate foods that may harm you during a flare, do so only if you've been on CBD for a few months and have not adjusted the dosage of the product you use.

I know how difficult it is to live with your symptoms, and how much CBD has benefited my symptoms, but only you know if CBD is right for your lifestyle. I hope at the very least I was able to provide you with the knowledge you need to approach its use with as much efficacy as possible to maximize its potential ability to help you in the way that you need. Go forth with bravery, always, to face the challenges we alone can see, and know that you are not alone.

Remember always: our disease is invisible, but we are not. We deserve to be more than spectators in our lives. We did not ask to prove our bravery, but we do so simply by living with our condition every day.

Be well, be strong, be brave.

Resources For CBD Use

1. Check Your's State's Current Laws

https://medicalmarijuana.procon.org/states-with-legal-cannabidiol-cbd/

The current status of CBD products across all 50 U.S. states, where its laws differ from the federal legalization of CBD oil. Some products other than oil may still not be legal in some states.

2. Check Leafly Marketplace

https://www.leafly.com/news/lifestyle/how-to-find-right-site-to-buy-cbd-online

The Leafly application can be downloaded to your phone to show you the closest dispensaries to you in your area, as well as those retailers' products before you visit. However, this particular article provides more on the how and where to buy for consumers who want to be more informed about CBD availability to them. It also provides information on assistance programs and marketplace websites where you can compare brands within your state or by product type.

3. Check Amazon

https://www.amazon.com/cbd-products/s?k=cbd+products&page=3

If you have Amazon Prime and want to add CBD to your regimen without paying for shipping, Amazon does sell certain brands. You can choose to subscribe and save if you plan to use these brands for chronic symptoms.

4. Do Your Own Research

https://medicalmarijuana.procon.org/questions/should-can-nabidiol-cbd-be-a-medical-option/

For more information about leading opinions on CBD, both for and against, visit procon.org and type in "CBD" to become more acquainted with the facts. Though I've attempted to provide you with data that supports its use, CBD is not FDA approved or regulated, nor is there a wealth of research into its effects on patients long-term. Naftali and colleagues are often held up as leaders into the study of medical cannabis, yet their studies are not irrefutable proof that CBD or medical marijuana should be touted as a supplement specifically for IBD. Their sample sizes of patients are quite small, and the studies often fail to follow up for a significant amount of time after the study is completed. It is up to you to make the choice you think is right for you.

5. Find Online Communities and Current Events

https://badgut.org/information-centre/a-z-digestive-topics/cannabis/

If you want explore the medicinal uses of cannabis, including CBD, badgut.org has detailed information about the Endocannibinoid System and its relationship to IBD. The site is also a place to find out more about your experiences, whether you're trying to find a specialist or connect with other ostomates. It's a one-stop shop for all of the latest you need to know and resources you can use to improve your access to quality healthcare.

References

Ahmed, W., & Katz, S. (2016). Therapeutic Use of Cannabis in Inflammatory Bowel Disease. Gastroenterology & hepatology, 12(11), 668–679.

Ananthakrishnan AN, Gainer VS, Cai T et al. (2013). Similar risk of depression and anxiety following surgery or hospitalization for Crohn's disease and ulcerative colitis. Am J Gastroenterology;108:594–601.

Ardizzone, S., Cassinotti, A., Manes, G., & Porro, G. B. (2010). Immunomodulators for all patients with inflammatory bowel disease?. Therapeutic advances in gastroenterology, 3(1), 31–42. https://doi.org/10.1177/1756283X09354136

Bergamaschi, M. M., Queiroz, R. H., Chagas, M. H., de Oliveira, D. C., De Martinis, B. S., Kapczinski, F., Quevedo, J., Roesler, R., Schröder, N., Nardi, A. E., Martín-Santos, R., Hallak, J. E., Zuardi, A. W., & Crippa, J. A. (2011). Cannabidiol reduces the anxiety induced by simulated public speaking in treatment-naïve social phobia patients. Neuropsychopharmacology : official publication of the American College of Neuropsychopharmacology, 36(6), 1219–1226. https://doi.org/10.1038/npp.2011.6

Capasso, R., Borrelli, F., Aviello, G., Romano, B., Scalisi, C., Capasso, F., & Izzo, A. A. (2008). Cannabidiol, extracted from Cannabis sativa, selectively inhibits inflammatory hypermotility in mice. British journal of pharmacology, 154(5), 1001–1008. https://doi.org/10.1038/bjp.2008.177

Dahlhamer JM, Zammitti EP, Ward BW, Wheaton AG, Croft JB.

(2015). Prevalence of Inflammatory Bowel Disease Among Adults Aged ≥18 Years. MMWR Morb Mortal Wkly Rep 2016;65:1166–1169. DOI: http://dx.doi.org/10.15585/mmwr.mm6542a3external icon

Dannels, N. (2018). CBD Is The Best Treatment Option For Your Battle Against IBD. https://cannabidiol360.com/cbd-for-ibd/

Farraye, Francis A MD, MSc, FACG1; Melmed, Gil Y MD, MS, FACG2; Lichtenstein, Gary R MD, FACG3; Kane, Sunanda V MD, MSPH, FACG4 ACG Clinical Guideline: Preventive Care in Inflammatory Bowel Disease, American Journal of Gastroenterology: February 2017 - Volume 112 - Issue 2 - p 241-258 doi: 10.1038/ajg.2016.537

Fakhoury M, Negrulj R, Mooranian A, Al-Salami H. (2014). Inflammatory bowel disease: clinical aspects and treatments. J Inflamm Res. 7:113-120
https://doi.org/10.2147/JIR.S65979

Hueting WE, Buskens E, van der Tweel I, Gooszen HG, van Laarhoven CJ. Results and complications after ileal pouch anal anastomosis: a meta-analysis of 43 observational studies comprising 9,317 patients. Dig Surg. 2005;22:69–79

Hwang, J. M., & Varma, M. G. (2008). Surgery for inflammatory bowel disease. World journal of gastroenterology, 14(17), 2678–2690. https://doi.org/10.3748/wjg.14.2678

Irving, P.M., Iqbal, T., Nwokolo, C., Subramanian, S., Bloom, S., Prasad, N., Hart, A., Murray, C., O Lindsay, J., Taylor, A., Barron, R., Wright, S. A Randomized, Double-blind, Placebo-controlled, Parallel-group, Pilot Study of Cannabidiol-rich Botanical Extract in the Symptomatic Treatment of Ulcerative Colitis, Inflammatory Bowel Diseases, Volume 24, Issue 4, April 2018, Pages 714–724, https://doi.org/10.1093/ibd/izy002

Kafil, T. S., Nguyen, T. M., MacDonald, J. K., & Chande, N. (2018). Cannabis for the treatment of ulcerative colitis. The Cochrane Database of Systematic Reviews, 2018(2), CD012954. https://doi.org/10.1002/14651858.CD012954

Katz, S., Lichtenstein, G. R., & Safdi, M. A. (2010). 5-ASA Dose-Response: Maximizing Efficacy and Adherence. Gastroenterology & hepatology, 6(2 Suppl 3), 1–16.

Knights, D., Lassen, K. G., & Xavier, R. J. (2013). Advances in inflammatory bowel disease pathogenesis: linking host genetics and the microbiome. Gut, 62(10), 1505–1510. https://doi.org/10.1136/gutjnl-2012-303954

Mawdsley, J. E., & Rampton, D. S. (2005). Psychological stress in IBD: new insights into pathogenic and therapeutic implications. Gut, 54(10), 1481–1491. https://doi.org/10.1136/gut.2005.064261

Melamede R. (2005). Cannabis and tobacco smoke are not equally carcinogenic. Harm reduction journal, 2, 21. https://doi.org/10.1186/1477-7517-2-21

Mjoseth, J. (2015). NIH researchers reveal link between powerful gene regulatory elements and autoimmune diseases. National Human Genonme Research Institute. https://www.genome.gov/news/news-release/NIH-researchers-reveal-link-between-powerful-gene-regulatory-elements-and-autoimmune-diseases

Naftali T, Bar-Lev Schleider L, Dotan I, Lansky EP, Sklerovsky Benjaminov F, Konikoff FM. Cannabis induces a clinical response in patients with Crohn's disease: a prospective placebo-controlled study. Clin Gastroenterol Hepatol. 2013;11(10):1276–1280

Nienke Z Borren, Grace Conway, John J Garber, Hamed Khalili, Shrish Budree, Himel Mallick, Vijay Yajnik, Ramnik J Xavier, Ashwin N Ananthakrishnan, Differences in Clinical Course, Genetics, and the Microbiome Between Familial and Sporadic Inflammatory Bowel Diseases, Journal of Crohn's and Colitis, Volume 12, Issue 5, May 2018, Pages 525–531, https://doi.org/10.1093/ecco-jcc/jjx154

Osterman, Mark T MD, MSCE1; Sandborn, William J MD2; Colombel, Jean-Frederic MD3; Peyrin-Biroulet, Laurent MD4; Robinson, Anne M PharmD5; Zhou, Qian PhD5; Lewis, James D MD, MSCE1 Crohn's Disease Activity and Concomitant Immunosuppressants Affect the Risk of Serious and Opportunistic Infections in Patients Treated With Adalimumab, American Journal of Gastroenterology: December 2016 - Volume 111 - Issue 12 - p 1806-1815 doi: 10.1038/ajg.2016.433

Singh Singh, A., Al-Khoury A., Kurti, Z., Gonczi, L., Golovics, P., Kohen, L., Afif, L., Wild, G., Seidman, E., Bitton, A., Bessissow, T., Lakatos, P. P570 The burden of anaemia remains significant over time in patients with inflammatory bowel disease at a tertiary referral centre, Journal of Crohn's and Colitis, Volume 14, Issue Supplement_1, January 2020, Page S480, https://doi.org/10.1093/ecco-jcc/jjz203.698

Sunil Samuel, MBBS, PhD, Steven B. Ingle, MD, Shamina Dhillon, MD, Siddhant Yadav, MD, W. Scott Harmsen, MS, Alan R. Zinsmeister, PhD, William J. Tremaine, MD, William J. Sandborn, MD, Edward V. Loftus, Jr, MD, Cumulative Incidence and Risk Factors for Hospitalization and Surgery in a Population-based Cohort of Ulcerative Colitis, Inflammatory Bowel Diseases, Volume 19, Issue 9, 1 August 2013, Pages 1858–1866, https://doi.org/10.1097/MIB.0b013e31828c84c5

Targownik, Laura E MD, MSHS1; Singh, Harminder MD, MPH1; Nugent, Zoann PhD1; Bernstein, Charles N MD1 The Epidemiology of

Colectomy in Ulcerative Colitis: Results From a Population-Based Cohort, American Journal of Gastroenterology: August 2012 - Volume 107 - Issue 8 - p 1228-1235 doi: 10.1038/ajg.2012.127

Tresca, A. (2020). Differences Between Ulcerative Colitis and Crohn's Disease. https://www.verywellhealth.com/understand-the-differences-between-cd-and-uc-1943108

Zimmerman (2019). CBD For IBD: Current Research Into Effectiveness. Healthline.com. https://cannabidiol360.com/cbd-for-ibd/